Evidence-Based
Mental
Health Care

Commissioning Editor: Michael Parkinson
Project Development Manager: Clive Hewat
Project Manager: Frances Affleck
Designer: Erik Bigland

Evidence-Based
Mental
Health Care

Simon Hatcher

Senior Lecturer in Psychiatry
University of Auckland, Auckland,
New Zealand

Rob Butler

Consultant in Old Age Psychiatry
Waitemata Health, Auckland,
New Zealand

Mark Oakley-Browne

Professor of Rural Psychiatry
Monash University, Victoria,
Australia

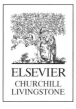

ELSEVIER
CHURCHILL
LIVINGSTONE

EDINBURGH LONDON NEW YORK OXFORD PHILADELPHIA
ST LOUIS SYDNEY TORONTO 2005

ELSEVIER
CHURCHILL
LIVINGSTONE

First published 2005

ISBN 0443073066

British Library Cataloguing in Publication Data
A catalogue record for this book is available from the British Library

Library of Congress Cataloging in Publication Data
A catalog record for this book is available from the Library of Congress

Notice
Medical knowledge is constantly changing. Standard safety precautions must be followed, but as new research and clinical experience broaden our knowledge, changes in treatment and drug therapy may become necessary or appropriate. Readers are advised to check the most current product information provided by the manufacturer of each drug to be administered to verify the recommended dose, the method and duration of administration, and contraindications. It is the responsibility of the practitioner, relying on experience and knowledge of the patient, to determine dosages and the best treatment for each individual patient. Neither the Publisher nor the authors assumes any liability for any injury and/or damage to persons or property arising from this publication.
The Publisher

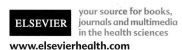

your source for books,
journals and multimedia
in the health sciences
www.elsevierhealth.com

The
publisher's
policy is to use
**paper manufactured
from sustainable forests**

Printed in China

Preface

The purpose of this book is to introduce the ideas of evidence-based practice to mental health practitioners so that they in turn can better help the people who come to see them. It is based on a course that two of us (S.H. and M.O.B.) taught at the University of Auckland to mental health clinicians. To date, most books on evidence-based practice have focused either on internal medicine or been written solely for a medical audience. We wanted to produce a book which was useful for mental health clinicians from a variety of professional backgrounds who are involved in direct patient care. We did not want to write just another book on critical appraisal. Instead we wanted to set evidence-based practice in a broader mental health context and describe some of the peculiarities of practicing in an evidence-based way within mental health. The importance of this approach is demonstrated by the fact that major professional organisations in mental health are now assessing critical appraisal skills as part of their examinations. (The Royal College of Psychiatrists and The Royal Australian and New Zealand College of Psychiatrists both test these skills in their exams.)

In writing this book we would like to acknowledge the work of David Sackett and others from McMaster who have been pioneers in the field of evidence-based medicine, and whose ideas are given another outing in this book. Also we would like to thank Christopher Cates for permission to use his diagram illustrating NNT. Finally thanks to the 'A' team for on-water discussions, the team in Liaison Psychiatry at North Shore Hospital for tolerating our absences, and Lyndy Matthews for support, provocation and reading the initial chapters.

'The fact that an opinion has been widely held is no evidence whatever that it is not utterly absurd; indeed in view of the silliness of the majority of mankind, a widespread belief is more likely to be foolish than sensible.'

Bertrand Russell: *Marriage and Morals* (1929)

Contents

1

Introduction – Why evidence-based mental health care?

People deserve it

Evidence-based mental health care exists because people who consult mental health practitioners deserve it. They have an ethical and often a legal right to know the answers to such questions as 'What evidence is there that this treatment will help me?', 'What is going to happen to me?' and 'What caused this?'. Practitioners need to be equipped to collaborate with patients to answer these questions. Evidence-based mental health care is a transparent process which equips patients and practitioners with powerful tools to address important questions of therapy, prognosis, diagnosis and etiology. It is an aid to making decisions about mental health care but is not sufficient in itself for guiding decision making, as this also depends on values and available resources. However, it does help to make such values explicit and can inform arguments about where resources should be directed. It is also effective for highlighting where there are gaps in knowledge and where the research effort should be directed. How different values are taken into account is particularly challenging in mental health care, as those of the wider society, the patient and their family may be widely divergent. Evidence-based mental health care does not provide easy answers to such problems, but it does provide transparency to the decision-making process. In our experience, the process is often as useful as the specific content. An alternative term that some may prefer is 'research-enhanced health care',[1] which emphasizes that evidence-based medicine was developed 'to encourage practitioners and patients to pay due respect – no more, no less – to current best evidence in making decisions.'

In many ways, it is easier to say what evidence-based mental health care is not. It is not an ivory-tower exercise carried out by academics. If it is to have any use at all it should be useful to clients and workers in a variety of settings. It is definitely not an exercise in statistics. Some basic understanding of chance and probability is useful, but the concepts are more

1

important than the mathematics. As a general rule, the more complicated the statistics, the less clinically useful the information! It is not cookbook health care where every patient comes with a set of instructions. We can be guided by what other people have experienced, but every clinical encounter is unique. It is not an attempt to drive out feelings from mental health care to be replaced by purely biological therapies.

The problems of the size of the literature and variations in mental health care

Another argument for evidence-based mental health care is for managing the enormous and growing mental health literature. In 2001, there were over 23 000 articles published on mental disorders and indexed in Medline. To keep up with this literature would mean reading over 60 articles a day. The problem is compounded by the fact that only about a third of the literature that is written gets indexed in Medline, meaning that the true number of articles published each year in the world on mental health topics is likely to be around 60 000. Furthermore, the rate of increasing information is increasing. Figure 1.1 shows the number of articles indexed under the term 'mental disorders' in Medline for the 20 years from 1981 to 2001. The time taken for the literature relevant to mental health care to double in size is about 18 years, which means that in a professional lifetime the amount of literature on mental health care will have increased fourfold. The tools of evidence-based medicine should help you and your clients select high-quality articles to read that are relevant to your situation. Probably more importantly, the tools help you decide what not to read.

Secondly, there is the problem of the variability of health care, which includes mental health care provision. It can often seem that the treatment a client gets depends on who they see rather than the problem they present with – a bit like a lucky dip. This can be a problem even

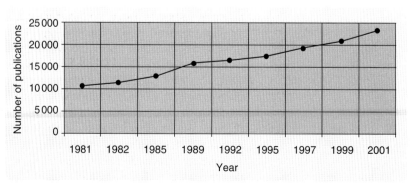

Fig. 1.1 The growth in mental health literature.

Box 1.1 Why evidence-based mental health care?
Ethically, people deserve to have the best available answers to questions such as 'What will help me feel better?'
Allows decision processes to become more transparent.
Offers useful tools to clinicians and patients.
Helps to identify a lack of resources.
Highlights gaps in knowledge.
Enables people to get the best from a huge amount of information.
Identifies the variability in mental health care delivery.

within the same organization. Kramer et al.[2] reported a study of over a 1000 patients enrolled in six different psychiatric clinics in the United States. A similar proportion of patients in each clinic were diagnosed as being depressed on various rating scales. However, the proportion of depressed patients who were offered antidepressants varied from 39% to 72%. Similarly, the mean number of psychotherapy sessions varied between the sites from four to nine, and there was no relationship between the number of psychotherapy sessions and the decision to prescribe antidepressants. The differences did not seem to be accounted for by clinical variables such as the level of functional impairment, which was similar across all sites. Paying due regard to the evidence may make going to a clinician less of a game of chance for the client.

The nature of evidence

The dictionary definition of evidence is 'the available facts, circumstances, etc. supporting or otherwise a belief, proposition, etc. or indicating whether or not a thing is true or valid'.[3] As the definition suggests, evidence comes in a variety of forms. When providing health care, this means that evidence may take the form of randomized controlled trials or it may be the wisdom of traditional cultural healers. However, in both these situations, evidence-based health care provides tools for deciding on the validity of their claims, their relevance for the client in front of you, and their importance. Particular caution needs to be applied to evidence based solely on an individual's experience and authority, whether they are a professor in a university or an indigenous healer, as mental health care is replete with examples of therapies and theories based on such evidence that have proved disastrous for patients.

Terminology notes

The language of research is confusing (a situation which is familiar to anyone who has studied psychotherapy). Students find themselves confused, (this is acceptable as it provides an impetus to find things out), and authors will use the same words to mean different things and different words to mean the same thing. For this reason throughout this text we have included notes on the terminology used in research, definitions, and examples of what we mean by the words we use. A good reference book that addresses this issue is, 'A Dictionary of Epidemiology' fourth edition, edited by John M. Last, Oxford University Press 2001. ISBN 0-19-514169-5

Problems with evidence-based mental health care

Feasibility

At the start of our course on evidence-based mental health care we ask the class what they think are the barriers to this approach. A common answer focuses on feasibility. Practitioners feel that they don't have access to resources, they aren't trained in this approach, and if they are, they find it hard to maintain their skills. Most importantly they say they do not have the time to practice in such a way. Formal research on the barriers to implementing evidence-based medicine has found that inadequate time to search for the information, failure of the resource to answer the question, difficulty formulating the question, difficulty in selecting a search strategy, and uncertainty about when to know when to stop searching for information are all important.[4] We hope this book will go some way to addressing these concerns.

Restricted to doctors

Most mental health research has been undertaken by doctors, published in doctors' journals, and read by doctors. This has been changing over the last few decades with a growing number of studies undertaken by nurses and an increasing number of publications aimed at nurses and other mental health professionals. The journals *Evidence-Based Nursing* and *Evidence-Based Mental Health* are aimed at or include nonmedical professionals. Many nursing interventions are being systematically defined and tested in trials. New therapies such as family interventions or compliance therapy for people with schizophrenia have been systematically evaluated and are being implemented by nurses and other nonmedical professionals. The model used for introducing these treatments aims at training interested professionals from different centers who then return to become trainers on a local basis.

Problems with health research governance

Cultural bias

More fundamentally, students identify problems with ownership of the evidence and biases in the research agenda – what is sometimes referred to as health research governance. Most health care research that is published focuses the problems of North Americans and Europeans. At a global level, only 10% of total spending on health research is used to investigate diseases that account for 90% of the global disease burden (the so-called '10/90 gap'). This is starkly illustrated by the fact that of the 1233 drugs that reached the global market between 1975 and 1997, only 13 were for tropical diseases that primarily affect the poor in undeveloped countries.[5]

Focus on drug treatments

As well as a focus on 'Western' diseases, there is also a preoccupation with drug treatments. In the major medical journals, 62% of randomized controlled trials focus on pharmacological interventions (with the noticeable exception of the *BMJ* where only a third of randomized controlled trials were on pharmacological treatments).[6] Of the 100 articles about treatment published in the *British Journal of Psychiatry* in 2001, 53% were on drug treatments, 19% on psychotherapies, 2% on both, and 25% on other topics (mainly service issues). Even within the psychopharmacology literature there are problems with the design and reporting of trials that distort the research database. Remarkably, between 89% and 98% of comparative drug studies funded by pharmaceutical companies show results that favor the funding companies product. Such sponsored research usually also demonstrates that the sponsored product causes less harm than its rivals. Safer[7] has described 13 discrete ways in which the design and reporting of such trials can be modified to demonstrate comparative superiority of one product over another.

Sex bias

There is also the issue of sex bias. In the field of addictions research, Brett[8] found that only 34% of the subjects included in the leading addiction journals in 1990 were female. This is a considerable improvement on previous reports which found that only 8% of the subjects in alcohol treatment studies between 1972 and 1980 were female. Researchers would provide a reason for using all female samples, but no reason for using male-only samples, implying that the male experience is the norm.

Age bias

Most research in mental health has involved people of working age. Often, studies have excluded people over the age of 50, 55, or 65 years old. There are a number of differences between younger and older people, which mean that treatments that work for younger people may work less well or be more harmful in the elderly. Older people are often not as efficient at metabolizing drugs, they have more medical illnesses that can be exacerbated by treatments, and they take more medications that can cause interactions. An example of excluding older people from research has occurred in electroconvulsive therapy (ECT). Despite the widespread use of ECT for older people with severe depression, in whom it is often considered a safer treatment than drugs, elderly people have been under-represented in trials. A systematic review of ECT for the depressed elderly only identified three relevant trials, all of which had methodological shortcomings.[9]

Agenda owned by researchers not consumers

It is also clear that consumers' research agendas vary from professional researchers. Tallon,[10] using osteoarthritis as an example, found that 76% of published and unpublished studies on intervention covered drug or surgical treatments whereas only 40% of patients identified researching such treatments as a priority. In contrast, 21% of patients thought education and advice should be given priority in research, whereas only 3% of published studies covered these areas.

Publication bias

Another problem is publication bias. Authors are less likely to submit, and editors are probably less likely to publish, articles which show negative results – for example, articles which don't show a difference in effectiveness between treatments are less likely to be published. This means that the research database is likely to contain articles that show results only in one direction. In some cases, pharmaceutical companies will actively try to prevent negative results from being published. The *New York Times* reported the case of a company that tried to block publication of a study that showed its HIV vaccine was not effective and threatened the researchers with US$7 million damages if they did publish.[11]

A related problem is the multiple publications of the same positive study in different journals, often under different lead authors. An extreme example of this is quoted by Duggan et al.[12] where one study on the effectiveness of olanzapine has been reported in 82 separate publications.

Strategies to address the problem of publication bias include searching for unpublished studies, using statistical tests (for example, funnel plots) to check for publication bias, and requiring all new trials to be registered when they are started (rather than when they are published).[13]

The advantage of an evidence-based approach is that at least all these distortions of the health care research database become transparent (Box 1.2).

Box 1.2   Problems with evidence-based mental health care

Clinicians do not feel they have access to resources.

Clinicians do not feel sufficiently trained to find and evaluate the literature.

Most studies focus on males of working age in the USA and Europe.

Most studies are about drug treatments.

Consumers are not involved in identifying areas to be researched.

Publication bias can results in positive results being more likely to be published than negative ones and multiple publications of positive findings.

The alternatives to evidence-based mental health care

When considering the problems of evidence-based mental health care it is also worth asking the question, what is the alternative? Mental health care provides many examples where ineffective therapies have been advocated that lack evidence for their effectiveness and have been adopted seemingly on the enthusiasm and authority of their promoters. Below are three examples of mental health treatment or ideas about etiology based mainly on the clinical experience of enthusiastic practitioners.

1. Lobotomy: an example of non-evidence-based treatment

Lobotomy was a procedure where a sharp instrument, like an ice pick, was pushed into the patients' frontal lobes via the orbital cavity. This was used to destroy nerve fibers with the result that the patient became more tranquil.

> I have also been trying out a sort of half-way stage between electroshock and prefrontal lobotomy on some of the patients. This consists of knocking them out with a shock and while they are under 'anesthetic' thrusting an ice pick up between the eyeball and the eyelid through the roof of the orbit actually into the frontal lobe of the brain and making the lateral cut by swinging the thing from side to side. I have done two patients on both sides and another on one side without running into any complications, except a very black eye in one case. There may be trouble later on but it seemed fairly easy, although definitely a disagreeable thing to watch.[14]

However, the price paid for this was a loss of personality, judgment, social skills, and disinhibition. At the peak of its popularity in the late 1940s lobotomy was being performed on more than 5000 patients a year in the United States. The initial evidence for the effectiveness of this operation was based on a series of 18 patients of whom only three were reported in any detail.[15] The question arises, how did this treatment, which is hard to defend ethically let alone on grounds of effectiveness, become so popular? In part, the answer is that doctors and patients were desperate to find a cure for intractable mental illnesses, so virtually any treatment would do. Just as importantly, an American psychiatrist Walter Freeman said it was a 'good thing' and actively promoted it personally and through an uncritical popular press. He invited to his academic presentations journalists whom he had briefed beforehand. He travelled extensively promoting the treatment. His biographer Elliot Valenstein wrote, 'On one five-week summer trip that year [1951], he drove 11 000 miles with a station wagon loaded, in addition to camping equipment, with an electroconvulsive shock box, a Dictaphone, and a file cabinet filled with patient records, photographs, and correspondence; his surgical instruments were in his pocket'.[16] (On this particular trip four patients died after surgery.) The point for this text is that a dubious and mostly ineffective treatment with significant side effects became popular largely because of an individual's authority and belief in the treatment.

2. The schizophrenogenic mother: a cause which wasn't

'A schizophrenic is always one who is reared by a woman who suffers from a perversion of the maternal instinct.' This quote from John Rosen, an American psychiatrist, encapsulates the concept of the schizophrenogenic mother, an idea that was prevalent in psychiatry for about 40 years from the 1930s.[17] The original idea was that schizophrenia was a socially based phenomenon that provided the theoretical basis for the psychoanalytical treatment of the disorder (despite Freud's biological conceptualization of the disorder). This led to the notion that it was mothers who were to blame for schizophrenia, especially those mothers who, 'wear men's clothes, try for commanding positions in business, and prefer not to care for their own children but hire nurses to play the role of makeshift mother. We also know that with the gratification of a perverted maternal drive, both the object and the one who exploits the object suffer'.[17] The evidence for this came mainly from small case series of selected patients with no control groups. Some researchers went further and, in early examples of what would now be called qualitative research, went to live in the patients' homes to observe the dynamics only to be outraged by the patients' mothers request that the (male) researcher help with the housework, which was used to demonstrate the mothers' schizophrenogenic emasculation of men.[18] When control groups were used and factors such as education and social class were accounted for, the schizophrenogenic mother concept was not supported, and over the space of 15 years disappeared from the literature. It had been allowed to thrive partly due to the lack of any contrary evidence, the highly selected sampling of a few cases, and the authority of the people promoting the idea.

3. Prolonged sleep therapy, psychic driving, and depatterning

Prolonged sleep therapy, psychic driving and depatterning (or brainwashing by any other name) mark one of the low points in psychiatry's history. Here, a president of the American Psychiatric Association and the World Association of Psychiatrists, Professor Ewan Cameron, received money from the CIA to provide treatment to depressed patients where the patients would be put into a chemically induced coma for several days, sometimes given ECT, and played repetitive tapes that were supposed to cure them of their depression.[19] Despite there not being a shred of evidence to support this as an effective treatment, it was allowed to continue and actively encouraged by the US government via the CIA, as they were interested in applying the results of this treatment to brainwashing prisoners of war from Vietnam. The patients treated by Professor Cameron have now taken legal action against the CIA, resulting in extensive documentation of this episode. There are many lessons to be learned from this sad story, but for the purposes of this book the lesson is that bad things can happen when the authority of respected individuals is used to justify therapeutic interventions in the absence of any other evidence for the treatment's effectiveness.

Other examples from the history of psychiatry include insulin coma therapy (the initial report on this therapy didn't even mention the number of patients treated) and malarial fever therapy.

The growth of evidence-based mental health

The first randomized controlled trial in mental health involved the treatment of 67 depressed British outpatients in 1955.[20] They were randomized to receive reserpine, an active ingredient of the plant rauwolfa serpentine, or a placebo, 'dummy tablets identical in appearance and almost indistinguishable in taste'. Of the 54 patients who completed the trial, there was no difference between the two groups on the doctor's and patients' ratings of outcome. Following this there was a wait until 1965 for the next randomized controlled trial in mental health, which again was of depression and compared imipramine, ECT, phenelzine, and placebo.[21] This study, done by the Medical Research Council in the UK, showed that phenelzine was not as effective as imipramine and ECT. The correspondence that followed is revealing and replicates many of the modern arguments about evidence-based medicine. 'There is no psychiatric illness in which bedside knowledge and long clinical experience pays better dividends; and we are never going to learn how to treat depression properly from double blind sampling in an MRC statistician's office'.[22] The irony is that the doctors (this was the 1960s and there were no nondoctors in the correspondence columns) who opposed this early example of evidence-based medicine were the proponents of aggressive psychiatric physical treatments such as insulin coma therapy and high doses of drugs. They used the arguments of the primacy of clinical experience and their authority to justify giving these treatments despite evidence to the contrary. The reply to William Sargant's letter, quoted above, by Bradford Hill is still relevant:

Unfortunately, as one of the patients in the bed I feel more than a trifle depressed while – partly at my expense – he gains his knowledge and his long clinical experience. I would have hoped that the process of learning might be a little less long if it were supported by the experimental method and attitude of mind. The statistician's office, needless to say, merely provides an experimental design upon which to hang the skilled clinical observation that must characterise any form of inquiry into therapeutic efficacy. There is no question of replacing valuable clinical observations by a series of mathematical symbols. Those who think so have the myopia of Don Quixote: they mistake the scaffold for the house.[23]

In the modern era, evidence-based medicine was consolidated and named in 1992 by a group of researchers and clinicians at McMaster

University in Canada.[24] Since then, interest has grown exponentially. Users, clinicians, managers, and politicians have all realized that evidence-based mental health care offers a way of improving the standards of mental health care.

Summary

Evidence-based medicine (or research-enhanced clinical care), exists to give clinicians and clients the tools to answer important questions about their care. The main barriers to practicing in this way involve issues of feasibility and problems with ownership and governance of the health research agenda. However, the history of mental health care is replete with examples of evidence-free treatments where patients have suffered as a result of the enthusiasm of others.

Evidence-based mental health care involves attitudes, skills, and behaviors. The set of attitudes involves a willingness to be open-minded and questioning about interventions; a willingness to collaborate with consumers to involve them in the process and incorporate their values in the decision-making process; and the acceptance that research can and should influence clinical practice. The skills involve knowing what are the important questions to ask, the process of answering them, and how or whether the answers are used in clinical practice. This is mainly the focus of critical appraisal. The behaviors involve a process of managing yourself to keep up-to-date with the literature, to answer clinical problems using an evidence-based approach and to incorporate evidence-based mental health care into everyday practice.

Adopting an evidence-based approach to care should make the enthusiastic application of treatments of dubious effectiveness less likely to happen in the future and enable consumers to receive the best care possible.

Patients, clients, and consumers

What to call people who attend mental health services is an issue. Some argue that the term patient is demeaning and disempowers people, while others argue that using the terms client and consumers is akin to treating health care as a commodity like washing powder. In this book we have generally used the terms patients, clients and consumers interchangeably without applying any value judgments to these terms. For what it is worth most (but by no means all) people who attend mental health services seem to prefer to be called patients.[25]

References

1. Devereaux PJ, Guyatt GH. Physicians' and patients' choices in evidence based practice. BMJ 2002; 324:1350.
2. Kramer T, Daniels AS, Zieman GL, et al. Psychiatric practice variations in the diagnosis and treatment of major depression. Psychiatric Services 2000; 51:336–340.
3. Oxford English Reference Dictionary. Oxford: Oxford University Press; 1996.
4. Ely JW, Osheroff JA, Ebell MH, et al. Obstacles to answering doctors' questions about patient care with evidence: qualitative study. BMJ 2002; 324:710–717.
5. Global Forum for Health Research. Available: *www.globalforumhealth.org* 3 Jan 2003.
6. Egger M, Bartlett C, Jüni P. Letters. BMJ 2001;323:1253.
7. Safer DJ. Design and reporting modifications in industry-sponsored comparative psychopharmacology trials. J Nerv Ment Dis 2002; 190:583–592.
8. Brett PJ, Graham K, Smythe C. An analysis of specialty journals on alcohol, drugs and addictive behaviours for sex bias in research methods and reporting. J Stud Alcohol 1995; 56:24–34.
9. Van der Wurff FB, Stek ML, Hoogendijk WL, Beekman ATF. Electroconvulsive therapy for the depressed elderly (Cochrane Review). In: The Cochrane Library, Oxford: Update Software, Issue 2, 2003.
10. Tallon D, Chard J, Dieppe P. Relation between agendas of the research community and the research consumer. Lancet 2000; 355:2037–2040.
11. Hilts PJ. Company tried to block report that its HIV vaccine failed. New York Times 1 Nov 2000.
12. Duggan L, Fenton M, Dardennes RM, et al. Olanzapine for schizophrenia (Cochrane Review) In the Cochrane Library, 1999.
13. Gilbody SM, Song F. Publication bias and the integrity of psychiatry research. Psychol Med 2000; 30(2):253–258.
14. Freeman W. History of psychosurgery. Unpublished manuscript, Himmelfarb Health Science Library, George Washington University.
15. Moniz E. Prefrontal leukotomy in the treatment of mental disorders. Am J Psych 1937; 93:1379–1385.
16. Valenstein E. Great and Desperate Cures: the Rise and Decline of Psychosurgery and other Radical Treatments for Mental Illness. New York: Basic Books; 1986:229.
17. Rosen J. Direct analysis: Selected papers. New York: Grune and Stratton; 1953.
18. Karon BK, Rosberg J. Study of the mother–child relationship in a case of paranoid schizophrenia. Am J Psych 1958; 12:522–523.
19. Thomas G. Journey into Madness: Medical Torture and the Mind Controllers. London: Corgi Books; 1989.
20. Davies DL, Shepherd M. Reserpine in the treatment of anxious and depressed patients. Lancet 1955; ii: 117–120.
21. Report to the Medical Research Council by its Clinical Psychiatry Committee. Clinical trial of the treatment of depressive illness. BMJ 1965; 1:881–886.
22. Sargant W. Antidepressant drugs (letter). BMJ 1965; 1:1495.
23. Hill AB. Reflections on the controlled trial. Ann Rheum Dis 1966; 25:107.
24. Sackett DL, Straus SE, Richardson WS, et al. Evidence-Based Medicine. How to Practise and Teach EBM. 2nd edn. Edinburgh. Churchhill Livingstone; 2000.
25. McGuire-Snieckus R. Patient, Client or Service User? Psychiatric Bulletin 2003; 27:305–308.

2

Formulating answerable questions

Evidence-based medicine is an important tool for solving clinical problems. It can also help the clinician give the best answers possible to patients. The first step to solving a clinical problem or answering a patient's question is to ask a clear question. Although that may sound easy, and with practice it can be, clinicians often need a framework to devise useful questions. This chapter describes how to formulate questions that you can answer. We outline three scenarios and look at how questions for each scenario can be framed. Later chapters describe how to go about answering them.

Important questions

The types of questions that clients and clinicians are often interested in are questions such as: 'What is wrong?' (diagnosis), 'What caused it?' (etiology), 'What is the best treatment?' (therapy), and 'What is going to happen?' (prognosis). Other questions are often about meaning and explanation, such as 'Why did it happen to me?', 'Why now?' and 'What does it mean for me and my family?'. Questions about meaning are closely related to clinical questions. 'Why did it happen to me?' and 'Why now?' are questions about etiology. The patient is trying to make sense of what has happened and the clinician can use evidence to help. 'What does it mean for me and my family?' is a question about outcome.

Formulating questions

To ask clear questions, we need to break the question into separate parts:

1. The patient or clinical problem.
2. The intervention of interest. Here the intervention is defined in broad terms as anything that the patient has happen to them – for example, it may be a treatment, exposure to a risk factor, or completion of a rating scale or other diagnostic test.

3. The comparison intervention if relevant.
4. The outcome that is of interest to the patient.

This is often abbreviated to **PICO** – Patient or population of interest, Intervention, Comparison, Outcome. The fifth and most important part of the problem is how to apply the answer in a clinical setting incorporating the patients' values, needs and wants.

Any clinical encounter may generate many questions. For an example, consider the following vignette:

A 35-year-old woman goes to a hospital emergency department after cutting her wrists. She is well known to the emergency department staff, having been there many times before, with similar injuries. She has been diagnosed as having a borderline personality disorder. She was sexually abused in her childhood.

'What is wrong?' (diagnosis) question.

The Patient	In women with borderline personality disorder
The Intervention	A rating scale that can be used by nonmental health staff
The Comparison if relevant	Not using a rating scale
The Outcome	To diagnose depression

'What caused this?' (etiology) question.

The Patient	In women with borderline personality disorder
The Intervention	Being sexually abused in your childhood
The Comparison if relevant	Compared to not being sexually abused
The Outcome	Contributes to the onset of the borderline personality disorder

'What will help?' (therapy) question.

The Patient	In women with borderline personality disorder
The Intervention	A psychological intervention
The Comparison if relevant	Compared to usual treatment
The Outcome	Decreases the frequency of self-harm

'What will happen?' (prognosis) question.

The Patient	In women with a borderline personality disorder
The Intervention	Does not attend therapy
The Comparison if relevant	Compared to attending therapy
The Outcome	Predicts a high risk of eventual suicide

'Why me?' (etiology) question.

The **Patient**	In people who deliberately self-harm
The **Intervention**	Women aged under 30
The **Comparison** if relevant	Compared to women over 30
The **Outcome**	At greater risk of a borderline personality disorder

'What does it mean for me and my family?' (meaning) question.

The **Patient**	In women with a borderline personality disorder
The **Intervention**	Attending family therapy
The **Comparison** if relevant	Compared to attending usual therapy
The **Outcome**	Predicts less family breakup

The advantage of asking questions in this way is that it helps to focus on a particular aspect of the patient's presentation that is of relevance to the patient and to our need to know. It also helps to focus search strategies in electronic databases. Clinicians often find it helpful to have some structure around which to form questions (Box 2.1).

Background questions

When faced with a clinical scenario there are numerous questions that may arise. This is particularly the case in mental health where almost all the clinical situations we face are complex. Some of these will be to do with the underlying psychological or physiological basis of a condition; for example, 'What is borderline personality disorder?' Sackett et al.[1] describe questions that ask for general knowledge of a condition as background questions. These questions usually start with a simple

---

Box 2.1   Questions that patients and their carers might ask

What is wrong? (diagnosis)

What else could it be? (differential diagnosis)

What tests are helpful? (diagnostic tests)

What caused it? (etiology)

Could it have been found sooner? (screening)

What will happen? (prognosis)

What treatments work? (therapy)

What prevents it? (prevention)

What does it mean for me and my family? (meaning)

questioning word (what, how, when, or why) followed by the disorder. Other background questions might include: 'what causes borderline personality disorder?', 'how common is borderline personality disorder?', and 'when do people with borderline personality disorder first present?'

Foreground questions

As clinicians become more familiar with and knowledgeable about a disorder, they tend to ask more detailed questions, called foreground questions. These questions have the four PICO elements, that is, Patient, Intervention, Comparison, and Outcome. In the 'what is wrong?' question, the foreground question is about using a depression rating scale to improve the diagnosis. The question has become more informed and more specific.

Why ask questions?

Patients may have questions for you, and questions may help you solve clinical problems. Asking questions helps a clinician identify areas they are not sure about. It is better to be explicit about areas of lack of knowledge than to bluff or hide your ignorance. Identifying an area of uncertainty is the first positive step towards identifying the answer. By asking questions as you work, it helps to use your learning time in areas that are directly clinically relevant. Patients may raise many of the pertinent questions themselves. These may offer research questions at a later date, and offer important teaching opportunities. Asking questions is rewarding for the clinician because it raises novel material and keeps the clinician curious.

Which questions to ask?

Given that there will always be more questions than time to answer them, we need to find a way to prioritize our questions. Key questions to help are 'what is most important to the patient?', 'what question is most feasible to answer in the time available?', and 'which is the question most likely to recur where I work?' Sometimes it is difficult to put the key question into words. In this case it is worth stepping back from the client and going through the core questions around diagnosis, therapy, etiology, and prognosis and asking either 'what don't I know?' or 'what is the key feature of this person's presentation?' Having identified the core clinical issue, we can build the question by filling in the component parts of the PICO question.

Looking at possible answers

Having found something that appears to answer a problem, we need to ask three questions:

- Is it true?
- Is it important?
- Is it relevant?

These questions are not mutually exclusive. A study may be true; in other words, its conclusions may be valid and believable, but the conclusions may not be important or relevant to you or your patients. Similarly, a study may produce important conclusions that are hard to believe because of the way the study has been done. Therefore, if the answer to *any* of these questions is 'no,' then we can discard that study and find something that better suits the clinician and their patients' needs. The guides to critical appraisal that occur in the rest of this book follow this structure and provide us with powerful tools to answer these three key questions.

Alternatives to PICO

Another commonly used acronym (used by Rod Jackson) is **PECOT** – which stands for the **P**opulation or patient; the **E**xposure of the patients to an intervention; the **C**ontrol group that may be exposed to a different intervention; the **O**utcome that we are interested in; and the **T**ime course over which the outcomes occur. This is useful for reminding the clinician that the time course of outcomes is often very important. Many interventions are tested over relatively short periods such as six weeks, whereas patients may be interested in how they will be in six months time or longer.

Exercises

Exercise 1

A 28-year-old woman presents to mental health services ten days after the birth of her first baby. She has experienced some auditory hallucinations and delusions about a global catastrophe. She has become increasingly distressed by these experiences and her husband is also concerned. The patient has had no contact with mental health services in the past and there is no family history of any psychiatric disorder.

Write foreground questions, using the PICO format, for each of the following types of questions: diagnosis, etiology, therapy and prognosis.

Exercise 2

A 23-year-old man was admitted to an acute psychiatric unit because voices were telling him to kill himself. He has a history of smoking cannabis. He is diagnosed as having schizophrenia.

Write foreground questions, using the PICO format, for each of the following types of questions: diagnosis, etiology, therapy and prognosis.

Answers

Exercise 1

Background questions for this vignette include 'What is post-partum psychosis?', 'How does post-partum psychosis present?' and 'What causes postpartum psychosis?'. A clinician unfamiliar with postpartum psychosis will understandably ask these sorts of questions. More experienced clinicians may make foreground questions by identifying a possible cause (first pregnancy) and formulating a question around that. The answers to these questions may also help the patient in their search for why it has happened to them.

These are some of the questions we came up with:

'What is wrong?' (diagnosis) question.

The **Patient**	In women with postpartum hallucinations and delusions
The **Intervention**	An abdominal ultrasound
The **Comparison** if relevant	Compared to a history and blood tests
The **Outcome**	Improves the diagnosis of delirium

'What caused this?' (etiology) question.

The **Patient**	In postpartum women
The **Intervention**	In their first pregnancy
The **Comparison** if relevant	Compared to subsequent pregnancies
The **Outcome**	More likely to suffer a postpartum psychosis

'What will help?' (therapy) question.

The **Patient**	In women with postpartum psychosis
The **Intervention**	Risperidone
The **Comparison** if relevant	Compared to haloperidol
The **Outcome**	Reduces the severity of the symptoms

'What will happen?' (prognosis) question.

The **Patient**	In women with postpartum psychosis
The **Intervention**	Having a supportive family
The **Comparison** if relevant	Compared to not having a supportive family
The **Outcome**	Decreases the likelihood of them having a psychotic illness not linked to pregnancy

Exercise 2

In this scenario, background questions are 'What is schizophrenia?', 'How does schizophrenia present?' and 'When do people with schizophrenia present?' The foreground examples we have chosen should help distinguish between a psychosis induced by smoking cannabis and schizophrenia.

Some of the questions we asked were:

'What is wrong?' (diagnosis) question.

The **Patient**	In a person who is psychotic
The **Intervention**	Cannabis intoxification
The **Comparison if relevant**	An acute episode of schizophrenia
The **Outcome**	Associated with auditory hallucinations

'What caused this?' (etiology) question.

The **Patient**	In a person with schizophrenia
The **Intervention**	Having a father with schizophrenia
The **Comparison if relevant**	Not having a first-degree relative with schizophrenia
The **Outcome**	Increases the likelihood of developing schizophrenia

'What will help?' (therapy) question.

The **Patient**	In a person with schizophrenia
The **Intervention**	Art therapy
The **Comparison if relevant**	No art therapy
The **Outcome**	Reduces the length of inpatient stay

'What will happen?' (prognosis) question.

The **Patient**	In a person with schizophrenia
The **Intervention**	Smoking cannabis
The **Comparison if relevant**	Not smoking cannabis
The **Outcome**	Increases the likelihood of rehospitalization

Reference

1. Sackett DL, Straus SE, Richardson WS, et al. Evidence-Based Medicine. How to Practise and Teach EBM. 2nd edn. Edinburgh Churchhill Livingstone; 2000.

3

Searching the mental health literature

There are several ways of searching for evidence. One of the most common is to ask other people. Other strategies include looking in textbooks, journals, and searching electronic databases. There are advantages and disadvantages to all these approaches (Box 3.1).

Asking other people

This could mean, for example, asking colleagues, discussions in peer review or in supervision. Asking colleagues has the advantage of being quick and convenient. However, there are several problems with asking other people. First, the information they have may be out of date. Second, their advice may be based on a different group of consumers than the ones you see. For example, clinicians confronted with psychotic patients in community mental health centers are likely to be managing people with schizophrenia or mania, whereas clinicians in a hospital liaison psychiatry service are much more likely to be treating delirium. Third, their evidence may be based on assumptions about underlying mechanisms, psychological, or physiological, rather than observations on the whole person. This has been termed 'reverse gullibility'[1] where knowledge of disease mechanisms or beliefs based on prior experience are given greater weight when making decisions than outcome data based on follow-up of real patients. As we have indicated in the previous

---

Box 3.1 Different ways of looking for evidence

- **Asking other people** – quick and convenient. Often biased and hard to check.

- **Looking in textbooks** – convenient but nearly always out of date. Biases present but not always transparent.

- **Searching electronic databases** – often inconvenient and time consuming. Requires some training. Difficulties compensated for by comprehensiveness of search and ability to retrieve only high-quality material.

---

chapter, to help evaluate all types of evidence you need to be able to answer three questions:

- Is it true (or valid)?
- Is it important?
- Is it relevant?

If the answer to any of these questions is negative, then the information isn't useful to you or your clients. Evaluating information from experts is no different. It is unlikely that in a conversation with someone you can assess the validity of a piece of information without checking the original source; however, you can assess importance and relevance. Therefore, three key questions to ask are:

- Will the information have a direct impact on outcomes that are important to my clients?
- Is the problem common or important in my practice?
- If the information is true, will it mean I have to change what I do?

A negative answer to any of these questions means that you can disregard the information. A positive response to these three questions means that you then have to assess the validity of the information. (Some authors refer to information that meets these criteria as POEMS – Patient Orientated Evidence that Matters.)[2] To assess the validity of the information, the next question you ask your expert colleague is:

- What is the reference or source of that piece of information?

And then there is no alternative to looking this up and assessing its validity!

Looking in textbooks

Textbooks are good for explaining concepts such as psychological mechanisms and subjects such as anatomy that do not change very much. They are not as good for looking up answers to clinical questions. There are two reasons for this: firstly, they are always out of date and, secondly, they have biases that are often hidden. Being out of date is a significant problem as the biomedical literature is large and grows almost exponentially (see Chapter 1 for a demonstration of this in mental health). The second problem is that chapters in textbooks are rarely written in a systematic and transparent way. It is usually unclear where authors derive the evidence for their recommendations from and what rules govern what evidence is included and what is excluded. The best textbooks have references that back up their recommendations and have a mechanism for regularly updating themselves – usually either via the Internet, through CD-roms, or through regular republication. An example of this is *Clinical Evidence*, (publisher BMJ Books *http://www.bmjbookshop.com*, see Box 3.2).

Box 3.2   *Clinical Evidence*

This book contains a continually updated summary of evidence about clinical interventions. For each condition, interventions are categorized as to whether there is evidence they are effective or not. The writers of each chapter search the literature and update every eight months. The section on mental health is published separately as Clinical-Evidence Mental Health. For example, in the chapter on depression, one of the questions is 'What are the effects of treatments?' The chapter lists a number of interventions as 'beneficial', the first being cognitive therapy. The systematic reviews and randomized controlled trials this is based upon are referenced. *Clinical Evidence* is published as a full text, a concise text, and an online version at *www.clinicalevidence.com*.

Searching electronic databases

The concept of a tiered approach to searching databases

Before describing the various electronic databases that are useful and accessible for mental health workers, we will introduce the notion of a staged or tiered search for information (Fig. 3.1). The reasons for this are that there are numerous electronic forms of databases that contain different types of information.[3] We have found that often students will jump straight into Medline to search for information rather than initially search other databases. These other databases may have relevant evidence already synthesized and appraised, which would save clinicians a lot of time.

Firstly, are those databases that summarize the evidence from several meta-analyses or collections of randomized controlled trials? These will have done the hard work of appraising the literature for you.

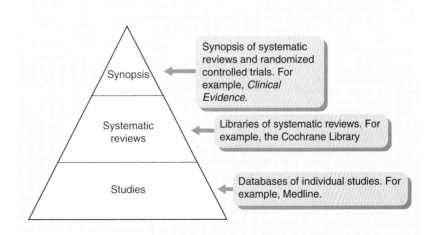

Fig. 3.1   A staged approach to searching electronic databases (adapted from Haynes[3], with permission from BMJ publishing).

For example, if you want to know whether bibliotherapy is helpful in treating depression, consulting the *Clinical Evidence* site (*http://www.clinicalevidence.com/*) will summarize the results of the numerous systematic reviews and randomized controlled trials and indicate the degree of certainty of the conclusions that can be reached. The disadvantages of these databases are that you usually have to subscribe to gain access and they address a limited range of disorders and treatments (although this is continually expanding).

If you cannot find useful information in those sites that produce a synopsis, then searching a database of systematic reviews is the next step. Systematic reviews are based on an explicit search for evidence, a transparent critical appraisal of the evidence found in the search, and a rigorous method of compiling and presenting the evidence. The gold standard for these is the Cochrane Database of Systematic Reviews, which is part of the Cochrane Library. These again will have done the work of appraising the validity and importance of the primary articles for you. However, they do not synthesize information from more than one systematic review, the reviews are often lengthy, making them hard to read in a timely manner, and currently they only address questions about the effectiveness of therapies. (A related database that has some marginal relevance to mental health issues is that of the Campbell Collaboration, which contains systematic reviews that focus on the effects of interventions in the 'social, behavioural and educational arenas' (*www.campbellcollaboration.org*).

The lowest tier in the hierarchy is the databases of primary studies such as Medline or PsycInfo. The advantage of these databases is that they are large, you can usually find something that seems applicable to you and the largest, Medline, is freely available on the Internet. The disadvantage is that finding clinically relevant articles can be difficult; searching skills have to be learned and practiced; and you are still left with the task of critically appraising the article.

Lastly, if the information is not available in the clinical databases then searching the Internet with Google or other suitable search engines is a useful way of finding evidence. The disadvantage of this is that it is often hard to assess the quality of information on the Internet, although there are guidelines on how to do this later.

The Cochrane Library
Background

The Cochrane Library is produced by the Cochrane Collaboration *http://www.cochrane.org/*. This is a worldwide organization that exists to produce systematic reviews on the effectiveness of interventions in health care. The name Cochrane comes from Archie Cochrane, a British medical researcher, who suggested that, because resources would always be limited, they should be used to provide equitably those forms of health care which had been shown in properly designed evaluations to be effective. (Also, as a result of his experiences as a prisoner of war, he recognized the relative unimportance of therapy compared to individuals' resiliency and capacity to heal without medical intervention.) The systematic reviews in the Cochrane Collaboration are produced by health care workers, consumers and researchers from around the world, loosely organized into about 40 Cochrane Review Groups. There are three review groups which are of most interest to mental health workers – the Cochrane Schizophrenia Group (*http://cebmh.warne.ox.ac.uk/csg/*), the Cochrane Depression, Anxiety and Neurosis Group (*http://www.iop.kcl.ac.uk/iop/ccdan/index.htm*), and the Drugs and Alcohol Group. There are also groups focusing on consumer issues, organization of care, as well as many other health care topics.

Access

Currently Internet access to the Cochrane Library is free for residents of Australia, England, Wales and the Irish Republic and Northern Ireland. Otherwise, access is by subscription or via hospital or educational networks. Abstracts of systematic reviews are freely available from the Cochrane Collaboration website. The Cochrane Library is updated twice a year.

Content

The Cochrane Library consists of several different databases. The three most likely to be useful to clinicians and consumers are:

- The Cochrane Database of Systematic Reviews (CDSR) – this contains two types of articles: complete systematic reviews on the effectiveness of health care interventions, and protocols for systematic reviews currently in progress.
- The Database of Abstracts of Reviews of Effectiveness (DARE) – this contains structured abstracts of systematic reviews that have not been done by the Cochrane Collaboration. The reviews have been appraised by the UK National Health Service Centre for Reviews and Dissemination.
- The Cochrane Central Register of Controlled Trials (CENTRAL) – this is a large database of over one-third of a million articles of controlled trials identified by the Cochrane Collaboration from multiple sources including electronic databases, handsearching of journals, and conference proceedings. The articles are not restricted by language.

Searching

Searching the Cochrane Library is fairly straightforward using a system of keywords. There is a help sheet for searching the Cochrane Library freely available from the Cochrane website.

Example

There is an example of a free abstract of a systematic review from the Cochrane Database of Systematic Reviews in Appendix A. Note that details of individual studies are not provided in these abstracts.

Medline
Background

Medline is the largest biomedical database, with over 12 million references to journal articles focusing on biomedical research and clinical topics including nursing and allied health from 1966 to the present. It is produced by the United States National Library of Medicine, which adds about 2000 articles every day (except Sundays and Mondays!).

Access

There are several different ways of accessing Medline. The most convenient is through PubMed which is freely available at many places on the Internet at *www.ncbi.nlm.nih.gov/PubMed/*.

An advantage of using PubMed to search Medline is that it is nearly always more up to date than other search tools. Medline can also be accessed through several commercial providers; one of the most common is Ovid, which is often used in educational institutions (other commercial providers are SilverPlatter and Aries Knowledge Finder).

A related free Internet access point also provided by the National Library of Medicine is Gateway at *http://gateway.nlm.nih.gov/gw/Cmd*. This searches several of the databases held by the Library, including Medline, using a single search engine. Other databases accessed by Gateway include OldMedline, Locatorplus, Medlineplus, AIDS Meetings, Health Services Research Meetings, and Space Life Sciences Meetings. The number of databases accessed by Gateway is intended to increase over time.

Content

Medline has a bias towards English language articles and journals published in the United States. For example, of 68 Spanish general medical journals only six are indexed in Medline.[4] It is important to recognize that not all biomedical and clinical journals are indexed in Medline – in fact it only contains about a third of the world's 12 000 biomedical journals. In the field of mental health, Medline indexes about half of the existing mental health journals.[5] There are some notable omissions; neither *Psychiatric Bulletin* from the UK Royal College of Psychiatrists, nor *Australasian Psychiatry* from the Australian and New Zealand College of Psychiatrists are included in Medline. Actually, this is not strictly true. There is one reference from Psychiatric Bulletin from 1992, 'Are psychiatric case notes offensive?', and this is included twice! This illustrates that one of the problems with such a massive database is that there will inevitably be mistakes, which will take the form of omissions and duplications. One study comparing handsearches of specialist journals (which included mental health journals) with the content of Medline found that 8% of the randomized controlled trials found by handsearching did not have a Medline record, despite these trials being reported in full in the handsearched journals.[6]

Searching

The second major issue with Medline is that with over 12 million records, finding what you want can be a challenge. To help with this on the PubMed website there is a tutorial on how to search the database. Searching is an acquired skill and to get good at it requires practice and familiarity with the search tool that is most convenient for you. To help searchers, all the records in Medline are indexed under several Medical Subject Headings or MeSH terms. Below is an example of a Medline record accessed through PubMed (Box 3.3). See Appendix B for complete abstract.

Box 3.3   Medline abbreviations

UI - Unique identifier (each Medline record has a unique number)

DP - Date of publication

TI - Title

AB - Abstract

AD - Address for correspondence

FAU - Full author name

LA - Language

PT - Publication type

CY - Country

MH - Mesh heading

SO - Source

The MeSH headings are prefixed by MH. This record is indexed under aged, antidepressive agents, depressive disorder, double blind method, drug therapy, female, human, lithium carbonate, male, recurrence, statistics, nonparametric and support, non-US Government. Some of the MeSH headings are followed by a / and further text; these are subheadings of the first term.

There are two important features of the MeSH indexing system. First is the 'focus' feature. In this record, three of the MeSH headings have an asterisk next to them – Antidepressive Agents/adverse effects/*therapeutic use; Depressive Disorder/*prevention & control; and Lithium Carbonate/adverse effects/*therapeutic use. The asterisks indicate that these indexing terms signify the major focus of this particular article. If you desire, you can restrict your search terms to just those that indicate a major focus.

The second important feature is that the indexing system is a hierarchical tree structure. The tree for depressive disorders is shown below. This indicates that the term depressive disorder is part of the category of mood disorders and that mood disorders is in turn part of the category of mental disorders. Underneath depressive disorder are four other indexing terms, each of which can be searched for specifically, which can be useful if all you are interested in is the subject of these headings. This tree structure has two important implications. Firstly, indexers are instructed to file articles under the most specific heading possible. Therefore, articles on postpartum depression are indexed under Depression, Postpartum *not* depressive disorders. To overcome this there is the ability to 'explode' a MeSH heading so that all terms underneath are automatically included. PubMed does this automatically unless you specifically turn it off. The disadvantage of exploding everything is that you can end up with large numbers of irrelevant headings. The second implication is that it is important to know the definitions or scope of

---

Box 3.4   MeSH tree for depressive disorder

All MeSH Categories

  Psychiatry and Psychology Category

    Mental Disorders

      Mood Disorders

        Depressive Disorder

          Depression, Involutional

          Depression, Postpartum

          Dysthymic Disorder

          Seasonal Affective Disorder

---

the MeSH headings and their relative position in the hierarchy. The MeSH term depressive disorder is defined as 'An affective disorder manifested by either a dysphoric mood or loss of interest or pleasure in usual activities. The mood disturbance is prominent and relatively persistent.' Note that psychotic depression is not included in this definition and it is actually a separate heading under mood disorders, Affective, Psychotic. This means that if you search for just depressive disorders, psychotic depression will be missed.

The last key feature of searching Medline is the ability to limit the search in important ways. One of the most useful is by type of publication. This is helpful as it introduces a quality filter so that if you have a large number of retrieved references about a therapy, for example, you can limit your search to references of higher likely validity by only retrieving those articles which cover randomized controlled trials.

Two particular problems with searching the mental health literature in Medline are the use of the terms depression and lithium. In MeSH terms, depression is not the same as depressive disorders! Depression is defined in MeSH terms as 'depressive states usually of moderate intensity in contrast with major depression present in neurotic and psychotic disorders'. Searching for depression does not yield the same articles as depressive disorders. Things are complicated in PubMed by the fact that the search engine automatically searches for the word you type in as both a MeSH heading and in the text of the title and abstract. This means that if you type in the word 'depression' you will get all the articles indexed under the MeSH term depression plus other articles which include the word depression anywhere in their title or abstract. (This may include articles that are really about the more severe depressive disorders, as well as articles that have nothing to do with mood disorders, such as papers on ECG ST depression in heart disease.) It is probably best to avoid using the term depression unless you really mean the milder forms of mood disorder.

The second mental health MeSH problem is with the drug lithium. Indexing for lithium is inconsistent. There are several MeSH terms that find articles on lithium – 'lithium' and 'lithium carbonate' are the two most common. Lithium refers to the lithium salt, and lithium carbonate to the mood-stabilizing agent. They are supposed to be mutually exclusive and appear at different places in the MeSH tree. However, in practice both are used to index articles on lithium in clinical use as a mood-stabilizing agent. For searches on the clinical use of lithium, all versions of the term should be used.

The importance of MesH headings is that they allow for precise searching and should help with finding relevant articles. There is no substitute for experience, practice, and advice when looking in massive databases like Medline; maintaining good relations with a medical librarian is fast becoming an important clinical skill. Success in finding answers to clinical questions seems to be related to experience in using Medline, the type of question (questions about prognosis and therapy are easier to answer than other types of question), and the ability to visualize spatial relationships among objects (Box 3.5).[7] (Interestingly, in this study attitudes towards computers and experience of computers were not related to successful searching.)

PsycINFO
Background

PsycINFO is a database of psychological literature produced by the American Psychological Association. It incorporates Psychological Abstracts, which is a monthly printed version of the database, and has

---

Box 3.5   Clinical queries in PubMed

In PubMed there is a facility to use specific search strategies for different types of clinical questions. This is called 'Clinical Queries' and is accessed on the left-hand tool bar in PubMed. The search strategies are for questions about therapy, diagnosis, etiology, and prognosis. You have the option of doing sensitive or specific searches. Sensitive searches retrieve large numbers of articles, most of which will not be relevant but you can be sure that most of the important articles have been found; specific searches retrieve fewer articles, which are more relevant but risks missing key papers.

The search strategies are based on a key paper by Haynes et al. published in 1994. Here, the authors used methodological terms to include articles which were likely to provide useful information for the type of question they addressed. However, there are several difficulties in relying on Clinical Queries for searching. First, the paper they are based on is now at least a decade out of date and there have been changes in how Medline indexes papers over the last ten years. Second, the Haynes et al. paper used general medicine journals as the gold standard to compare the accuracy of their searches – the search strategies in clinical queries are not mental health specific. Lastly, Clinical Queries cannot be used on other databases. However, the principle of searching based on methodological filters is sound and until further work is done on the best way of searching the mental health literature the search strategies in Clinical Queries are the best we have.

several products derived from it, including PsycLit, PsycFirst and ClinPsyc *www.apa.org/psycinfo/*.

Access

Access is by subscription either on a pay-as-you-go basis or annual payment. There are numerous private vendors who offer different types of access. Institutions often provide free access to individuals.

Content

At the time of writing there were just under 2 million articles in PsycINFO. Like Medline, PsycINFO contains abstracts and citations (not the full text of articles) but it also contains references to books, journals, dissertations, and reports (these form about a quarter of the database). It is updated weekly with nearly 77 000 citations added in 2001. There is considerable historical material in this database with, for example, the American Journal of Psychology being electronically indexed from 1887 to 1966.

Searching

Searching is by a system of Psychological Index Terms which are different from those used in Medline, although the principles remain the same.

EMBASE
Background

EMBASE is a pharmacological and biomedical database of journal citations published by Elsevier: *http://www.elsevier.nl/homepage/sah/spd/site/locate_embase.html*.

Access

Access is by subscription via several database vendors or free to individuals of institutions that have purchased access to the database.

Content

EMBASE focuses on pharmacological and biomedical subjects. It is big, with nearly 9 million references and about 450 000 references added annually. Because of its European origins, it is less likely than Medline to focus on English language articles. It is particularly strong on pharmaceutical studies reflected in the way it searches for drugs and their synonyms.

Searching

Searching is by indexing terms – EMTREE preferred terms – which are similar to but not the same as Medline (although there is considerable overlap). Despite its bias towards drug studies, EMBASE appears to be useful for nondrug therapies as well. For example, one study compared PsycInfo, Embase, and Medline in a search for randomized controlled trials of cognitive behavior therapy. The authors found that EMBASE was better than PsycINFO but not as good as Medline at finding relevant articles.[8]

CINAHL
Background

CINAHL (the Cumulative Index of Nursing and Allied Health Literature) is a United States bibliographic database covering the nursing and allied health literature.

Access   Access is by subscription or free to individuals who belong to institutions that have purchased access to CINHAL.

Content   The focus is on the nursing and allied health literature. The database contains references to journals, books, websites, newsletters, standards of practice, relevant US government publications, and patient education material. The database consists of about 750 000 records taken from about 1500 journals.

Searching   Searching is by CINHAL's own unique system of subject headings although these are similar to the MeSH headings in Medline.

                          There is also a physiotherapy database of systematic reviews and randomized controlled trials, PEDRO, at *http://www.pedro.fhs.usyd.edu.au/index.htm*, and an occupational therapy database of systematic reviews and randomized controlled trials at *http://www.otseeker.com/*.

Mental health literature on the Internet

The Internet is a good source of information for rare disorders, consumer perspectives, and a number of other resources such as rating scales. There are two difficulties, however. Firstly, the information available is constantly changing and growing, with new sites appearing and old ones not being updated. This means that any recommendations made here are likely to be out of date in a few years' time. Despite this, some of our favorite sites on evidence-based medicine are listed in Box 3.6.

Box 3.6 Useful web sites on evidence-based health care

http://www.nettingtheevidence.org.uk/ From the school of Health and Related Research at the University of Sheffield, UK. Excellent links to many EBM articles and resources.

http://www.jr2.ox.ac.uk/bandolier/ The home page of *Bandolier*, a web-based EBM journal from Oxford, UK.

http://www.library.unisa.edu.au/internet/pathfind/ebmed.htm#austcebhc From the University of South Australia in Adelaide, a friendly and well laid out site providing links and information about a wide range of evidence-based health care sites.

http://www.miart.co.uk/i-medicine.info/default.asp A UK-based site attractively laid out with links to useful EBM information and helpful practical information on topics such as running a journal club.

http://www.cebmh.com/ The centre for evidence-based mental health based in Oxford, UK.

Secondly, and more fundamental, is the problem of knowing what is high-quality information. There have been numerous attempts to come up with guidelines for discriminating high-quality medical sites from the rest.[9] One of the most commonly used is DISCERN, which is a 16-item questionnaire, freely available from the Discern website at *www.discern.org.uk*. The aim of this tool is to 'help users of consumer health information judge the quality of written information about treatment choices' that includes Internet websites. An alternative to appraising individual sites is to access health information via 'gateways' which open to sites that have already met some criteria of quality measured against a gold standard. Clearly there is an issue over what the gold standard is, but sites accessed by these gateways are generally of better quality than others. Examples of these gateways include Health on the Net, (*http://www.hon.ch/*), OMNI (*http://omni.ac.uk*), HeathInSite (*http://www.healthinsite.gov.au/*), Healthfinder (*http://www.healthfinder.gov/*), MedlinePlus (*http://medlineplus.gov/*), and the Canadian Health Network (*http://www.canadian-health-network.ca/*).

Exercises

Exercise 1

You are rung by a colleague who is seeing a 31-year-old woman with a history of alcohol abuse, self harm, and brief intense relationships. She says that the client has a diagnosis of borderline personality disorder. Your colleague is getting increasingly frustrated with attempts at managing this woman. Your colleague wants to know if you know of any effective psychological therapies for this woman. Create a four-part question based on this scenario. Do a literature search based on this question for the psychological management of borderline personality disorder.

Exercise 2

You are looking after a 25-year-old young man who has just recently experienced his first psychotic episode. His parents want him to have a CT scan. You're not sure that this is necessary because his clinical examination was normal. Construct a four-part clinical question around this scenario. Perform a literature search to find what evidence exists to support the value of CT scanning as a diagnostic tool in patients after their first episode of psychosis.

Exercise 3

A 28-year-old woman has recently been diagnosed as suffering from bipolar disorder. She has never had to be hospitalized for her disorder. She wants to know from you what her prognosis is. Do a literature search to discover what evidence is available on the prognosis of bipolar disorder for this woman.

Exercise 4

You are seeing a 35-year-old man with a ten-year history of alcohol dependence and abuse. He has a history of drunken driving and has lost work because of his alcohol abuse. He tells you that his father was an alcoholic and that this is why he also has a problem with alcohol. Do a literature search to find out what evidence exists which addresses the role a parental history of alcohol abuse plays in the etiology of alcohol dependence and abuse in male children.

Answers

Exercise 1

This is a question about treatment, so the question will go something like, 'In women with borderline personality disorder (the population) is a psychological therapy (the intervention) better than usual care (the comparison) in improving self harm, substance abuse and quality of life (the outcomes)?'

One way to go is to search Medline using PubMed. We opened Clinical Queries in PubMed, clicked on the therapy and sensitive buttons, and put in the term 'borderline personality disorder'. This retrieved over 350 articles, still a large number, but scrolling down the first page we hit gold with a Dutch study by Verheul et al. in the *British Journal of psychiatry* on a randomized controlled trial of dialectical behaviour therapy in borderline personality disorder. As this is a question on therapy, however, we may find that there are systematic reviews on this topic, so the Cochrane Library or *Clinical Evidence* may be useful. Going to the *Clinical Evidence* website and looking at the list of topics in the mental health section, there is currently no entry for personality disorders, so this is not useful. Searching for borderline personality disorder in the Cochrane Database of Systematic Reviews and the Database of Abstracts of Effectiveness (DARE) – both part of the Cochrane Library – we got seven and four hits, respectively. The references in the Database of Systematic Reviews weren't particularly helpful, but one of the hits in DARE was a systematic review of 'Psychotherapy for personality disorders' by Perry et al. which has the advantage that someone else has already done the work of gathering together and appraising studies relevant to our question. The only disadvantage is that this review is slightly out of date, having been done in 1999.

Exercise 2

This is a question about diagnosis. The question then is, 'In young men who have had a psychotic episode with no physical signs (the population) what value is a CT scan (the intervention) in detecting intracerebral causes of psychosis (the outcome)?' As this is not about therapy, the Cochrane Library and *Clinical Evidence* are of no value. Therefore, we searched PubMed using initially the term 'first episode psychosis' which yielded nearly 500 references. We then entered the term 'CT scan' which produced nearly 150 000 hits (PubMed automatically converted our term 'CT scan' into 'tomography, X-ray computed' [MeSH Terms] or 'Ct scan' [Text Word]). Combining these results yielded 12 hits, one of which from 1988 was on the utility of CAT scanning in first-episode psychosis by Battaglia. If we wanted to find a more recent study, then we could enter this study into a database called Science Citation Index, which searches forward in time by seeing which articles have cited a particular reference. It would be reasonable to assume that articles that had cited the Battaglia article would be close to the topic we are interested in. Entering this article on Science Citation Index shows that it has been cited in: Gen Hosp Psychiatry. 1988 Nov;10(6):398–401, Utility of the CAT scan in a first psychotic episode. Battaglia J, Spector IC.

Exercise 3

This is a prognostic question, so straight to Medline via PubMed. Using the clinical queries box, we entered 'bipolar disorder' and clicked on prognosis and sensitive search. This resulted in over 3000 hits, so we needed to somehow reduce this number. First we limited the search by making it adult, English language, and studies with abstracts. This reduced the number of studies to about 1600, so still too many. The next step was to limit this even further by selecting review articles which produced about 80 hits. However, scrolling through the studies, none was really what we were interested in. Therefore, we went back and looked at specific rather than sensitive studies plus bipolar disorder in the clinical queries box. This produced only 540 studies and scrolling through the first two pages we came across a study by Judd et al. on the long-term follow-up over 20 years of a cohort of bipolar I and bipolar II patients. This answer demonstrates the concept of 'limiting' searches and the difference between sensitive and specific approaches to searching (in this case 3000 studies versus 540 studies).

Exercise 4

This is a question about etiology. So again, because Medline is freely available via PubMed, we used that to search for evidence about this question. This resulted in over 700 hits. Now, these articles were about many causes of alcohol abuse, so we typed in the term 'genetics' (over 1 million hits) and combined this with our initial 700 hits which resulted in about 100 relevant articles. Scrolling through the first page, we came across a study by Finn et al. on the effects of familial risk, personality and expectancies on alcohol use and abuse published in the *Journal of Abnormal Psychology* in 2000.

References

1. Riffenburgh RH. Reverse gullibility and scientific evidence. Arch Otolaryngol Head Neck Surg 1996; 122:600–601.
2. Slawson DC, Shaughnessy AF. Obtaining useful information from expert based sources BMJ 1997; 314:947–949.
3. Haynes RB. Of studies, summaries synopses, and systems: the '4S' evolution of services for finding current best evidence. Evid Based Ment Health 2001; 4:37–38.
4. Marti J, Bon ll X, Urrutia G, et al. Identicacion y descripcion de los ensayos clinicos publicados en revistas espanolas de medicina general e interna durante el periodo 1971–1995. [The identification and description of clinical trials published in Spanish journals of general and internal medicine during the period of 1971–1995] Med Clin (Barc) 1999; 112(Suppl 1):28–34.
5. Taylor L, McDonald S, Adams C. Are you searching the right database? An example from mental health. 6th Annual Cochrane Colloquium Abstracts, Baltimore, October 1998.
6. Hopewell S, Clarke M, Lusher A, et al. A comparison of handsearching versus MEDLINE searching to identify reports of randomized controlled trials. Statist Med 2002; 21:1625–1634.
7. Hersh WR, Crabtree MK, Hickam DH, et al. Factors associated with success in searching MEDLINE and applying evidence to answer clinical questions. J Am Med Inform Assoc 2002; 9:283–293.

8. Watson RJ, Richardson PH. Identifying randomized controlled trials of cognitive therapy for depression: comparing the efficiency of Embase, Medline and PsycINFO bibliographic databases. Br J Med Psychol 1999; 72:535–542.

9. Darmoni, S J Haugh, M C Lukacs, B, et al. Quality of health information about depression on internet: Level of evidence should be gold standard. BMJ 2001; 322:1367.

4

What is the best treatment?

How do we know what is the best treatment for an individual? There are many ways of answering this question.[1] Firstly we could try an intervention in an individual patient and see if it works. The difficulty with this is that you only know in retrospect if the treatment is effective, which could be a problem with some lengthy psychotherapies or drug treatments and, secondly, it doesn't take into account the natural history of any disorder. After all the client may have improved without any intervention. Alternatively, you could identify a group of people with the disorder and treat some of them and not treat others. The difficulty here is that the groups may be different in some important respects that may influence whether treatment is effective. For example, if the question is, 'Does cognitive behaviour therapy improve symptoms in drug-refractory schizophrenia?', you could divide a group of people with drug-resistant schizophrenia in two and treat one group with cognitive behavior therapy while the rest get usual care. The difficulty here is that one group, for example, may have a significantly longer history and have more severe symptoms than the other group. This would clearly influence their chances of responding to any treatment. One way to get round this is to identify before doing the trial those factors which may influence treatment and ensure that they are evenly distributed between the two groups. The problem that arises here is with factors we don't know about, which influence treatment response. In the schizophrenia example it may be that particular personality traits we are unaware of are important in determining who responds to treatment. The way to avoid this problem of not knowing is to randomize individuals into the different groups. This ensures that by chance those factors which influence treatment we know about *and those we do not* are evenly distributed between the groups. This is the rationale for doing randomized controlled trials which, in most cases (the exceptions we'll describe later), are the best way of determining the effectiveness of different interventions.

What is a randomized controlled trial?

The ideal behind a randomized controlled trial is that the only difference between the groups in a trial is the treatment they get. Therefore, any change you see in the groups is due to the intervention. In other words, they strive to be like controlled experiments where all the different variables are held constant except one, the intervention, so that any differences at the end of the trial are due to the therapy. In real life this is not always the case and the critical appraisal of randomized controlled trials is essentially assessing the threats to this ideal. The participants in a randomized controlled trial are selected from a wider population and then randomly allocated to a treatment group and one or several comparison groups. Random allocation means that each individual should have the same chance of receiving all the possible treatments and that this chance is not influenced by what treatments other participants receive. The ways that individuals are randomized vary but can be as simple as having the allocation in concealed envelopes or as sophisticated as having a computer-generated random allocation (Fig. 4.1).

Problems with randomized controlled trials

Ethics

There are ethical problems concerning the treatment groups and the comparison groups. Some treatments or interventions are inherently harmful, and randomly allocating individuals to receive them would be unethical. For example, smoking is clearly harmful to health but it has also been suggested that it can prevent some forms of dementia. Randomly allocating people to smoke or not smoke would be difficult to justify to an ethics committee. In these circumstances the effects of an intervention would have to be studied by other methods; in the

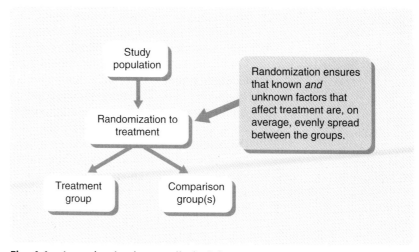

Fig. 4.1 A randomized controlled trial.

smoking example, probably by case–control or cohort studies. Similarly, it would be hard to justify treating the comparison group with a placebo or nothing if they had already been identified as suffering from a serious disorder. For example, if the study group consisted of individuals who were depressed and suicidal, it would be hard to ethically do a trial where one group got a treatment and the comparison group received no care.

Cost

Randomized controlled trials are financially expensive. Costs involve paying for the process of randomization, recruiting individuals, following them up, providing two or more different treatments and assessing the outcomes. Costs for doing such trials can run into millions of dollars.

Harm

Randomized controlled trials are not good at addressing the question of rare but important side effects. Because such adverse events are rare, they may not occur at all in an individual trial. An example is the association of suicide with selective serotonin reuptake inhibitors. While it is still not clear whether such an association really does exist, the answer is unlikely to be found by looking at individual randomized controlled trials, as suicide is such a rare occurrence. Typically, suicide occurs at a rate of 10 to 20 per 100 000 people, so it is unlikely that any trial will ever be large enough to find a significant difference in the rate of suicide between people treated with selective serotonin inhibitors and any comparison treatment. Other problems associated with detecting harm in randomized controlled trials is that researchers do not know what harms to look for; there may be a long delay between exposure to an intervention and any subsequent adverse outcome; harms may be measured in different ways in different trials; and adverse effects may be mistaken for symptoms of the original condition.

Critical appraisal of randomized controlled trials

Is the study valid?

Was the assignment of subjects to treatment randomized? Was the randomization concealed?

The first part of this question is to ensure that the participants really were randomized. Methods which appear random but which aren't are allocating people to treatment groups based on date of birth, time of presentation, or by the number on the patient's notes. The randomization list should also be concealed from the researchers doing the trial. This is to ensure that the researchers can't predict which treatment group the next subject will be allocated to. If they can, biases both conscious and unconscious may come into play. For example, the researchers may tend to put subjects with a good prognosis into the new treatment group, therefore maximizing any therapeutic effect. Returning to the cognitive behavior therapy in drug-resistant schizophrenia question, a recent study by Sensky et al.[2] specifically addressed this issue (Fig. 4.2). Here, 90 patients with schizophrenia, which was resistant to drug

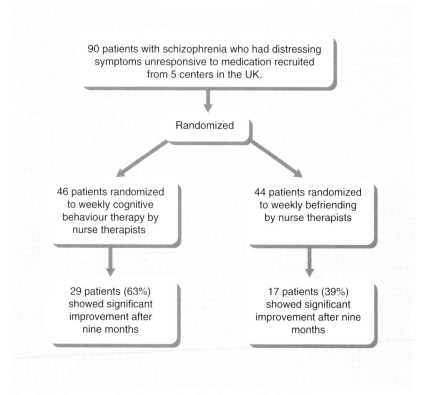

Fig. 4.2 An example of a randomized controlled trial – cognitive behavioral therapy for persistent symptoms in schizophrenia resistant to medication.[2]

treatment, were randomized to receive either cognitive behavior therapy or befriending delivered by nurse therapists. The cognitive behavior therapy focused on understanding the symptoms and methods to reduce the distress and disability caused by them, while the befriending involved sessions on neutral topics such as sport and hobbies. The paper states that the patients were randomized by 'simple randomization', which was performed independently of the research team. The authors don't state what they mean by 'simple randomization', but it is reasonable to assume that it was a procedure akin to tossing a coin where heads gets you into one group and tails into the other. It is easier to assess whether the randomization list was concealed, as the authors specifically state the researchers were independent from the people doing the randomization.

Was follow-up of patients sufficiently complete and long enough?

It is important that follow-up of patients is as complete as possible – the ideal is that all subjects who start a trial are included in the final results. This is because if we only include the patients who get to the end of the trial, and ignore people who drop out, this can distort the results and overemphasize the effect of therapy. Figure 4.3 shows what happens in a

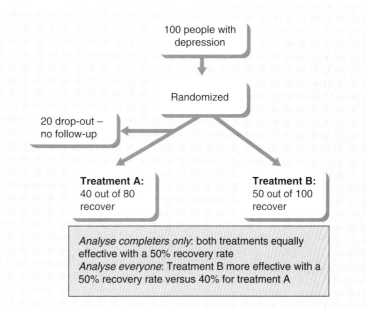

100 people with
depression

Randomized

20 drop-out –
no follow-up

Treatment A:
40 out of 80
recover

Treatment B:
50 out of 100
recover

Analyse completers only: both treatments equally
effective with a 50% recovery rate
Analyse everyone: Treatment B more effective with a
50% recovery rate versus 40% for treatment A

Fig. 4.3 The importance of complete follow-up in randomized controlled trials.

hypothetical situation where subjects are lost to follow-up in a trial comparing two treatments for depression. Here, 100 people with depression are randomized to one of two treatments, A or B. In the group receiving treatment A, 20 people do not complete the trial because of side effects or being unable to complete the treatment, but of the 80 who complete, 40 are recovered. In the group receiving treatment B, no one drops out but 50 recover. If we analyse the results just on who completes the trial, then the treatments are equally effective, but if we include the subjects who have dropped out we then see that treatment B results in recovery 50% of the time and A is less effective with a 40% recovery rate.

Drop-outs can seriously affect the validity of randomized controlled trials so that most leading journals won't publish trials with less than an 80% follow-up. In the schizophrenia and cognitive behavior therapy trial, although 15 patients failed to engage in therapy or only had minimal amounts, they were still followed up and accounted for at the end of the treatment trial – so, unusually, in this study the follow-up was a commendable 100%.

Additionally, the trial should be of sufficient duration to observe clinically important effects. If the study is too short, then it stands only a small chance of observing clinically important changes. For example, in the schizophrenia and cognitive behavior therapy trial, if it had only followed patients for a few weeks it would not be helpful clinically; in fact, it followed patients for nine months after treatment finished, which gives us some indication of how persistent any changes brought about by the treatment actually are.

Were the subjects analysed in the groups to which they were randomized?

The important issue here is that once patients are randomized they are then 'in' the trial and should be included in any analysis. This is regardless of whether after randomization they then refused to take their medication or take part in the therapy to which they are assigned. The analysis of all patients after randomization to their separate groups is called an 'intention-to-treat analysis'. The importance of this is that it preserves the benefits of randomization (people may refuse treatment after allocation for many reasons, some of which may be related to factors that affect treatment), and is more akin to clinical practice. As clinicians, we know that the process of agreeing to therapy is different from the process of starting therapy. We need to know what happens when we offer a treatment to someone that they are prepared to accept. It is of limited value to know what happens just to people who take the treatment if 90% refuse it after they have accepted it. (People may get worse or improve in between accepting and starting treatment.)

In the schizophrenia and cognitive behavior therapy study, it specifically states that an intention to treat analysis was carried out and the six patients who were unable to engage in therapy and the nine who ended treatment prematurely were included in the analysis. After reviewing the first three major critical appraisal questions, we can be reasonably sure that any results from this study are likely to be valid. There are also three further questions about treatment trials we could consider if we have time.

Were the researchers and patients blind to the treatment?

Researchers and patients can have strong feelings about which are the best treatments and this may bias any results. Bias may be introduced by, for example, introducing other treatments, differential reporting of symptoms or completion of outcome measures or influencing what patients report. The way to avoid these affecting the outcome of a trial is to find a way to make sure that neither the researchers nor the patients are aware of what treatment they are receiving – in other words to blind them to the treatment. If both the researchers and the patients do not know, then it is double blind, and if only one of them is unaware of the treatment, it is single blind. As with much of the language of research, the term 'blind' has been used in different ways[3] and authors are now encouraged to be transparent about who was aware of treatment allocation when reporting studies. Some drug trials will also attempt to assess how successful blinding was by asking clinicians and patients at the end of the trial if they can guess which treatment they were taking. The results of such a trial are more believable if the participants were unable to do so, as it demonstrates that the blinding was successful.

In the schizophrenia and cognitive behavior therapy trial a particular problem, which is common to all psychotherapy studies (and most surgical studies), is that the patients were clearly aware of what treatment they were getting – it was impossible to blind them. One way to partially get around this is to make sure that the researchers who do the assessment of outcomes are unaware of what treatment the patients received. In our example, the authors state that the assessors 'remained blind to each patient's assigned group throughout the study' and also that they were a different group from those who were providing the treatment.

Were the groups treated equally, apart from the different treatments?

The results of a randomized controlled trial will be more believable if, after the subjects are randomized, the different groups are treated equally in all respects apart from the intervention introduced by the researchers. The differential treatment of the groups may be apparent in the way that outcome data is collected or by one of the groups receiving supplementary treatment.

With the schizophrenia and cognitive behavior therapy study, it could be that any differences in the two therapies have been minimized because one of the groups received either extra medication or some other intervention. The authors measured drug use in the patients during the trial and found that 'similar proportions of patients had their drug dose increased during the study, or were given atypical antipsychotic drugs'.

Were the groups similar at the start of the trial?

The validity of the findings from a randomized controlled trial are increased if we know that the groups of subjects were similar at the start, especially in factors which may affect outcome. This is often the first issue that is reported in the results of any trial. If the groups were unequal in some important respects, we would look to see that this had been taken into account in the analysis of the results.

In the schizophrenia and cognitive behaviour therapy example, the two groups were similar in age, ethnicity, length of illness, number of admissions, and the presence of delusions and hallucinations.

Are the results of the study important?
What is the size of the treatment effect?

The issue here is that although studies may produce valid and statistically significant effects they may not be clinically important. To assess whether a valid finding is clinically important you need first, of all, clinical knowledge followed by some understanding of basic mathematics.

If a study finds an association between an intervention and an outcome, this can be due to four things: bias, confounding, chance, or it can be a true cause and effect (Box 4.1). This applies to all research designs but it is most useful to discuss it in relation to randomized controlled trials. The role of bias and confounding is assessed by the questions about the validity of a study. Chance is assessed by doing various statistical tests that tell you the likelihood of any observed outcome happening by chance. Clearly, if an outcome is unlikely to happen by chance we would consider such a finding significant. Conventionally, the threshold to be impressed by is a less than 1 in 20 likelihood of a finding happening by chance, usually expressed as $p < 0.05$. (This figure can change depending on how many statistical tests authors perform on their results. Clearly, the more tests are done the more likely it is that by chance a finding of $p < 0.05$ will occur. In these circumstances the threshold for significance is changed by applying what is known as the Bonferroni criteria).

Box 4.1   Bias and confounding

Bias This is defined as a systematic error in the design or conduct of a study which leads to a false association between an exposure and an outcome. Bias is usually introduced by the researcher (but unlike in normal usage doesn't imply prejudice). The prevention of bias is mainly through study design. Once it occurs it is hard to correct for and readers of studies need to consider the magnitude and direction of any bias and how it may have affected the results.

Confounding This occurs when an association between an exposure and an outcome is caused by a third factor independently related to the exposure and outcome. Unlike bias, it is normally due to complex inter-relationships between different exposures and outcomes in 'real-life'. For example, in the study of cognitive behavior therapy and schizophrenia, a confounding factor could be social class. Those who engage with and do well in the former may be of higher socioeconomic class. However people in a higher social class have more resources, so would be expected to have a better outcome of their schizophrenia. Here, social class could be related both to the likelihood of engaging in treatment and to a good prognosis for schizophrenia. Control of confounding occurs in the design of the study (randomization or matching, for example) and in analysis (multivariate analysis and stratification).

Reference: Sackett DL Bias in analytical research. J Chron Dis 1979:32;51–63.

Having established the roles that bias, confounding, and chance may play in a study, and being satisfied that they won't significantly distort the results, we can then pay attention to the importance of any effect. The size of any effect is usually expressed in one of two ways depending on whether the outcome is a continuous measure, such as a rating scale measure, or a dichotomous measure, for example, 'recovered' and 'not recovered'. The problem with continuous measures in mental health care is that, firstly, they make assumptions about the numerical properties of rating scales that often are not true and, secondly, it is hard for consumers and clinicians to know what they mean. For example, it is hard to know what an average reduction of 4 points on the Beck Depression Inventory really means in clinical practice – although this may well be a statistically significant result. For this reason, studies are increasingly reporting discrete outcomes in mental health, so for example in the schizophrenia and cognitive behavioral therapy study the authors decided that for patients to count as having had a good outcome they needed to reduce their scores on the comprehensive psychiatric rating scale (CPRS) by greater than 50% between the start of the study and at nine months.

There are several ways in which the size of any treatment effect can be described. In our example, 63% of patients had a greater than 50% improvement in their CPRS scores with cognitive behavior therapy compared to 39% with the same improvement who received befriending. The difference is 24% (63–39%), and 24% is 0.61 of 39%, so the relative improvement of cognitive behavior therapy compared to befriending is 0.61, (or 61% as a percentage). In other words, cognitive behavior therapy is 61% better then befriending. This is called the relative risk

Table 4.1 The different ways of expressing outcomes in clinical trials

	Outcome after 9 months		
	Number of people with a greater than 50% improvement in CPRS score	Number of people with a less than 50% improvement in CPRS score	Number of patients randomized
Cognitive behavior therapy	29	17	46
Befriending	17	27	44

- **Absolute risk of improvement after 9 months with cognitive behavior therapy:** 29/46 = 0.63 or 63%
- **Absolute risk of improvement after 9 months with befriending:** 17/44 = 0.39 or 39%
- **Relative risk:** 0.63/0.39 = 1.61
- **Relative risk improvement (RRI)** = 1.61–1 = 0.61 or 61%
- **Absolute risk improvement (ARI)** = 0.63–0.39 = 0.24 or 24%
- **Number needed to treat for nine months with cognitive behavior therapy compared to befriending to get one extra person better** = 1/0.24 = 4

(sometimes relative risk improvement or reduction depending on the direction of change). The disadvantage of this measure of change is that it does not take into account the magnitude of the risks it is comparing. For example, the relative risk is the same if befriending results in 3.9% of people improving and cognitive behavior therapy 6.3%; however, the clinical meaning is very different (Table 4.1). The relative risk can produce seemingly large improvements with only small differences in treatment, for example a change from 1% of people recovering to 1.25% of people produces a relative risk improvement of 25%.

Another way of expressing the result is the absolute risk reduction or improvement, which is the difference between the two outcomes, so that in our example the absolute risk improvement is 24%. If the results were 3.9% and 6.3% then the absolute risk improvement would be 2.4%, so this seems better than the previous relative risk. However, we can improve on the absolute risk by using its inverse, which provides a whole number and tells us how many patients we need to treat to get one extra good outcome compared to the control treatment – this is called the number needed to treat (NNT) and in our example is 100%/24%, which is 4.

How the results of trials are expressed can make a big difference as to whether clinicians, doctors, and managers are influenced by them. For example, in a review of this matter, McGettigan et al.[4] found that physicians were more likely to report a change in practice or treatment decisions if results were presented in terms of relative risk rather than absolute risk or NNT (see Table 4.2).

The number needed to treat can also be used to describe the adverse effects of treatment when it is referred to as the number needed to harm. The number needed to treat has two important properties. Firstly, it is a comparative measure. A treatment does not have an NNT in isolation; it is always in relation to some other intervention. Secondly, the NNT is described with a time period. The clinical meaning of an NNT can be

Table 4.2 Comparison of relative risk, absolute risk and NNT

Improved with treatment A out of 100 subjects	Improved with treatment B out of 100 subjects	Relative Risk Improvement	Absolute Risk Improvement	NNT
3	2	50%	1%	100
15	10	50%	5%	20
30	20	50%	10%	10
60	40	50%	20%	5
90	60	50%	30%	3

Note how the relative risk does not change with alteration of the absolute size of the treatment effect.

vastly altered by the time it takes to treat. For example an NNT of 4 over 2 weeks has a very different interpretation of an NNT of 4 over 2 years. To compare NNTs of treatments over different times it is necessary to convert them to the same duration, which can be any clinically meaningful time. For example, when comparing an NNT of 3 over 12 weeks to 5 over 6 months we can multiply 3 by 2 (as there are roughly 2×12 weeks in 6 months) to get an NNT of 6 over 6 months. Note that this makes the assumption that the improvement from the treatment is constant over time and does not, for example, occur all in the first few weeks.

Notwithstanding the advantages of NNTs, there are also some disadvantages (Box 4.2). First, the NNT is often defined as the number of people needed to treat to avoid one bad outcome. This causes problems because it is hard to explain the benefits of treatment by talking about the avoidance of bad outcomes. When discussing treatments with patients, we prefer to talk about the number of people needed to treat to achieve one extra good outcome compared to the alternative treatment (see later in this chapter). Second is the problem that the NNT makes the assumption that benefit from an intervention occurs uniformly over time. Strictly speaking, the results from a trial should not be extrapolated to time points beyond that considered in the study. Third, the NNT assumes that it does not vary for different levels of risk. This may not be true; for example, the more severe a depressive disorder, the more effective are physical treatments. There are bedside methods for adjusting different baseline risks, which we will describe in the next section on relevance. Next is the problem of expressing the results of meta-analyses and odds-ratios in terms of NNT, which can sometimes be misleading. Lastly, despite being supposedly easier to understand and more meaningful than other outcome measures, the limited evidence so far suggests that this may not be so. Kristiansen et al.[5] report a Danish study where members of the general population were asked to rate how likely they were to take a drug to prevent a heart attack. The authors varied the NNT when asking people their opinion and found it made no difference to their choice as to whether to take the medication. However, in this

---

Box 4.2 Problems with NNT

- Not all trials report NNTs.

- Sometimes hard to compare if subjects have different baseline risks.

- Should not be used to extrapolate beyond the time period of a study (unless it is reasonable to assume consistent benefits over time).

- Limited evidence suggest they don't make a difference to treatment decisions.

- Definitions confusing, concentrating on preventing bad outcomes, therefore hard to describe to patients.

- Can be misleading in meta-analyses or case–control studies.

---

study, other factors may have been important; in particular, the authors said that the drug only had few and mild side effects.

When reporting the results of a trial, no single statistic is sufficient in itself to help in decision making. The emphasis increasingly is on transparency of reporting clinical trial results so that consumers and clinicians can calculate results which are meaningful for their particular needs.

How precise is the measure of the effectiveness of treatment?

Randomized controlled trials are done using a study population recruited by the investigators. The study population in turn is part of a population of potential recruits for the study – the so-called experimental population. This population in turn is part of a reference population. These relationships are illustrated in Figure 4.4. The reference population is the group to which the researchers expect the results of any trial to apply.

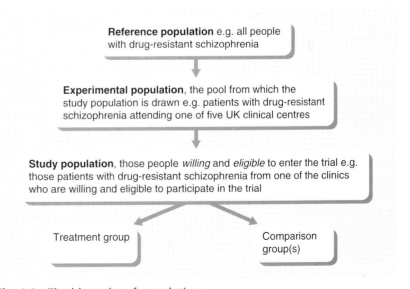

Fig. 4.4 The hierarchy of populations.

So in the schizophrenia and cognitive behavior therapy trial, the reference group is all people who suffer from schizophrenia with unremitting symptoms despite adequate drug treatment. The experimental population is the pool of people in whom the trial is conducted, so in this example they are people with schizophrenia with drug-resistant symptoms attending one of five clinical services in the UK. The study population is those patients from the experimental population who are willing and eligible to take part in the trial. The relationships between these different populations are important for questions about the relevance of a trial and the precision of any measure of treatment effectiveness. We will consider here questions about precision. It is clear that the study population is only a small subset of the reference population, which is all people with drug-resistant schizophrenia. If the study were done again using a different study population, the results would be unlikely to be exactly the same as the first study. If the study were repeated a third time on a different study population, then it is likely the results will be different once more, and so on. However, we would expect the results to be similar and spread around the 'true' result. Also, the larger the study population, in other words the closer in size it got to the reference population, the closer the result would be to the true outcome if we included everyone with the condition in the study. The measure of precision that we use is called the confidence interval and a working definition is, 'the range of values within which we can be 95% sure that the reference population value lies'. So in our schizophrenia example the absolute risk improvement is 24% with 95% confidence intervals between 4% and 44%, whilst the NNT is 4 with 95% confidence intervals between 2 and 23. What this means is that we can be 95% certain that the 'true' (reference) population value for the difference between the treatments could be as low as 4% or as high as 44%; similarly, we can be 95% certain that the 'true' population value for the NNT could be as low as 2 or as high as 23. There are three important characteristics of confidence intervals. Firstly, the larger the population the narrower the range, because as the size of the study population approaches that of the reference population the more likely any result will be closer to the true value for the reference population. Secondly, if the confidence intervals cross the point of no difference, the result could have happened by chance and is not statistically significant. Thirdly, the 'true' value is most likely to occur in the middle of a range of confidence intervals, as the probability of its occurrence through the range is described by a bell-shaped curve.

Are the results of the study relevant to our situation?

Is our patient so different from those described in the study that we can not apply the results?

The patients that we see are rarely identical to those described in a treatment trial. However, the differences between the patients described in the study and those seen by clinicians are usually quantitative rather than qualitative. In other words, while there may be, for example, a difference in the degree of responsiveness to therapy, it is unlikely that therapy will produce completely different outcomes to those described in a treatment trial. Examples of differences which may make a treatment trial inapplicable may be co-morbid conditions that make the treatment impossible to carry out, for example: significant thought disorder in people with schizophrenia may make cognitive behavior therapy impossible; different pharmacogenetics in different cultures may alter how drugs are metabolized which may render them ineffective; or different cultural styles of interpersonal attachment may affect the applicability of some psychotherapies. Because such occasions are rare, it is relatively unusual for treatment trials to be discarded at this hurdle.

Is the treatment feasible where we work?

Here we have to consider whether it is feasible to deliver the therapy in the health care setting where we work. In some settings there are restrictions on what medication is available and the provision and availability of trained therapists. For example, if access to cognitive therapists is restricted then it is unlikely that trials of cognitive behavior therapy in schizophrenia will be relevant to you and your clients (although having a trial that demonstrates the effectiveness of this therapy may make it easier for you to make a case for more funding for such treatment).

What are the potential benefits and disadvantages for our patient?

To recommend an intervention to a patient we need to know two things: first, the probability of different outcomes and, second, what value the patient (or as often occurs in mental health, the values of other people) places on these different outcomes. (This is no different from how we make most conscious decisions.) An exhaustive version of this is called decision analysis and is described in Chapter 11. The problem with decision analysis is that it is time consuming to use in routine clinical practice. A simpler process is incorporated in the last two critical appraisal guides about relevance. The first part of individualizing a treatment decision is therefore to calculate the probability of different outcomes for a patient. In this simple version we just use the most important outcomes – recovery versus no recovery, major harms versus no harms. In the schizophrenia and cognitive behavior therapy, there are no significant harms reported, so we can just use the clinical bottom line – significantly improved versus no significant improvement NNT of 4. We now need to estimate how quantitatively different our patients are from those in the trial. If we estimate that our patient is twice as hard to treat (because of chronicity, social class, or substance abuse issues for example), than the patients treated in the study then we double the NNT to 8. Similarly if we think the patient has an outcome that is probably twice as good as those in the study (possibly because of good social support or previous treatment response), then we half the NNT to 2. Although this may seem remarkably like flying by the seat of our pants, studies suggest that experienced clinicians may be quite accurate in estimating relative differences in baseline risks. More complicated ways of calculating the difference between the risks of individual patients and those in trials rely on examination of risks of subgroups of patients in large treatment trials; using clinical prediction rules to derive estimates; or using prognostic studies (or local databases) of similar patients. We can do similar calculations for the risk of being harmed.

A novel way of showing the risks and benefits of treatment is with pictures, an example of which we have shown in Figure 4.5. This is taken from Christopher Cates EBM website at *http://www.nntonline.net/* where the programme VisualRx is available to download. This programme quickly produces pictures that illustrate the effects of treatment. Figure 4.5 illustrates the potential benefits from cognitive behavior therapy in drug-resistant schizophrenia. With befriending (no active treatment), 39 out of 100 people improve; with cognitive behavior therapy an extra 24 out of 100 people improve.

What values does the patient or significant others place on the major outcomes for the treatment and can they be incorporated into decision making?

In many ways this is the least well explored part of the critical appraisal process. It is particularly difficult in mental health where there are often legal constraints on what can or should be done; there are many players in the decision-making process besides the patient; and the disorder itself may influence decision making and the values clients place on the different outcomes. None of these problems is unique to mental health, just more obvious than in other areas. There is a potential here for mental health to lead the way for other clinical disciplines in describing how to make individual health care decisions. There is no correct way of doing this, but there are several steps which most people agree on. First is a decision about who to involve in the decision-making process and to what degree do they want to be involved. Second is the description of the therapy with its associated potential benefits and harms. Third is the exploration of the patient's and important other's values about the potential outcomes. Last is the decision itself, which incorporates risks,

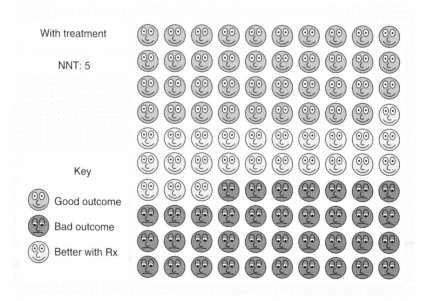

Fig. 4.5 VisualRx picture of the benefits of cognitive behavior therapy in schizophrenia.

benefits, and values. How expansive and thorough each step needs to be will vary with every clinical encounter. Clearly, offering someone ten sessions of cognitive behavior therapy for an anxiety disorder will be different from making a decision about a sex-change operation. Eliciting values can be by a variety of methods including time trade-off, standard reference gamble (described in the section on decision analysis), or by using a rating scale.[6] Incorporating these values into the decision-making process is less clear cut. Sackett et al.[7] describe a process called 'likelihood of being helped versus harmed'. Here, the patient is asked to estimate on a scale from 0 to 1 the values that they place on continuing to be unwell (that is the bad outcome that treatment is trying to prevent), and the value they place on any adverse event associated with the treatment. (If the treatment has no significant adverse effects, then the value placed on it is one.) The ratio of these two ratings gives a measure of how much a patient values improvement versus adverse effects. The ratio of the number needed to treat divided by the number needed to

---

Box 4.3 A note on psychotherapy (and surgical) randomized controlled trials

There are several challenges in carrying out psychotherapy trials that are shared with studies which attempt to assess the effectiveness of surgical interventions.

- First, there is the 'it's obvious it works, therefore we don't have to assess it' argument. For example, clinicians will argue that an intervention such as talking to people about traumatic events after a disaster or the removal of gall stones surgically is so obviously beneficial that there is no point in doing a randomized controlled trial to assess its efficacy. However, just because something is obvious does not mean it is true. For example, there are now several randomized controlled trials which indicate that talking to people about traumatic events after a disaster may make them more likely to develop post-traumatic stress disorder in the future.

- Second is the problem of operator skill. Different therapists/surgeons have different skills. This needs to be accounted for in clinical trials. The usual way of doing this in psychotherapy trials is to record the treatment sessions and see how closely the sessions met predefined criteria for skill often described in a treatment manual. If the treatment is described in a manual it is also more exportable to other settings.

- Third is the issue of blinding. Patients and therapists are rarely blind to the treatment they have delivered or received in psychotherapy/surgery trials. To minimize the bias this introduces, outcomes are usually assessed by researchers not involved in treatment who are kept blind to which group the patient was allocated.

One way forward for clinical disciplines where the drug metaphor of doing trials breaks down is to develop clinical databases of everyone entering treatment that can provide evidence on the effectiveness of therapy.

Reference: Black N. Developing high quality clinical databases BMJ 1997:315;381–382.

harm is then multiplied by this figure to produce a numerical measure of how likely they are to be helped or harmed by the intervention. This technique works with treatments with few only significant adverse effects but is less useful when there are multiple mild but possible harms. To our knowledge this way of presenting information and decision making has yet to be formally tested. An initiative that aims to improve the reporting of randomized controlled trials is the CONSORT statement[8] which is a set of guidelines for authors of such studies.

Exercises

For these exercises we will summarize a study and then ask questions based on that study.

Ockene JK, Adams A, Hurley T et al. Brief physician– and nurse practitioner–delivered counselling for high-risk drinkers. Does it work? Arch Intern Med 1999; 159: 2198–205 as summarized in Evidence Based Nursing 2000; 46: 3.

Design

Randomized (unclear allocation concealment), blinded (outcome assessors), controlled trial with 6 months of follow-up.

Setting

The setting was four primary care internal medicine sites at a university medical center in Massachusetts, USA.

Patients

There were 530 patients between 21 and 70 years of age (mean age 44 years, 65% men) who were scheduled to be seen at one of the primary care sites and who were high-risk drinkers (men who drank >12 drinks/week or binged on >4 drinks on at least one occasion in the previous month; or women who drank >9 drinks/week or binged on >3 drinks on at least one occasion in the previous month). Patients were excluded if they were pregnant, planned to move out of the area within 1 year, did not have a telephone, were already on an alcohol intervention programme, or had an Axis 1 psychiatric disorder. Follow-up was 91%.

Intervention

The 4 primary care sites (38 physicians and 8 nurse practitioners) were randomized to the intervention (n = 274 patients) or usual care (n = 256 patients). Physicians and nurse practitioners in the intervention group had 2.5 hours of training on the patient-centered alcohol intervention program. Patients in the intervention group received a health booklet with advice on general health issues and a 5–10 minute counselling session at the time of their routine visit. Patients in the usual care group received the same health booklet and were encouraged to direct any health questions they had to their physician or nurse practitioner. All physicians and nurse practitioners were encouraged to attend weekly conferences that included biannual presentations on managing patients with alcohol problems.

Main outcome measure   Change in alcohol use (weekly alcohol use and frequency of binge drinking episodes/month) at 6 months.

Main results   After adjusting for age, sex, and baseline alcohol consumption, patients who received the intervention had lower alcohol consumption than those who received usual care (mean reduction 5.8 vs. 3.4 drinks/week, $p = 0.001$). No difference existed for mean reduction in binge drinking episodes per month between patients in the intervention group and those in the usual care group (1.8 vs. 1.0, $p = 0.09$).

Conclusion   Brief counselling by a physician or a nurse practitioner as part of routine primary care reduced alcohol consumption by high-risk drinkers.

Questions

1. Is the study valid?
(a) Was the assignment of subjects to treatment randomized?
(b) Was the randomization concealed?
(c) Was follow-up of patients sufficiently complete and for long enough?
(d) Were the subjects analysed in the groups to which they were randomized?
(e) Were the researchers and patients blind to the treatment?
(f) Were the groups treated equally, apart from the different treatments?
(g) Were the groups similar at the start of the trial?

2. Are the results of the study important?
(a) What is the size of the treatment effect; what is the number needed to treat (NNT)?
(b) How precise is the measure of the effectiveness of treatment; what is the 95% confidence interval?

3. Are the results of the study relevant to our situation?
(a) Is our patient so different from those described in the study that we cannot apply the results?
(b) Is the treatment feasible where we work?
(c) What are the potential benefits and disadvantages for our patient?
(d) What values does the patient or significant others place on the major outcomes for the treatment and can they be incorporated into decision making?

Answers

1. Is the study valid?
(a) Yes, the assignment of subjects to treatment was randomized.
(b) No, how the allocation was concealed is not explained in the paper.
(c) Yes, there was a high rate of follow-up (91%) over a six-month period. However, it would be interesting to see if the brief counseling sessions continued to be effective at a longer follow-up point.
(d) Information not given.
(e) Yes, the outcome assessors were blind to treatment. The patients would have known which group they were in.
(f) Yes, both groups had usual care apart from the intervention.
(g) No, the researchers adjusted for age, sex, and baseline alcohol consumption.

2. Are the results of the study important?

(a) At six months, there was almost a two-fold adjusted mean reduction in weekly alcohol use for those who had received the intervention. An NNT is not given because the result is a continuous variable (number of drinks per week). However, the result could have been given as the proportion of people in each group who drank less than (say) 8 drinks a week – if that is felt to be an outcome that reduces harm.

(b) Information not given.

3. Are the results of the study relevant to our situation?

(a) Yes, the baseline level for high-risk drinking appears low and participants who were identified as high-risk drinkers may not have viewed themselves as such. The study excluded those who did not have a telephone, were already on an alcohol intervention program, or had a psychiatric disorder. These sampling issues may limit the generalizability of the study findings.

(b) Yes, the intervention is brief, although clinicians will need 2.5 hours of training and weekly conferences. There will be cost and resource implications.

(c) The potential benefit is reduced drinking and subsequent harm; there should be no major disadvantages for our patient.

(d) It is not clear what value the patients place on reduced drinking. However, the high rate of follow-up suggests the patients valued the study.

References

1. Streiner DL. Thinking small: Research designs appropriate for clinical practice. Can J Psych 1998; 43:737–741.
2. Sensky T, Turkington D, Kingdon D, et al. A randomized controlled trial of cognitive behavioural therapy for persistent symptoms in schizophrenia resistant to medication. Arch Gen Psychiatry 2000 Feb; 57:165–172.
3. Devereaux PJ, Manns BJ, Ghali WA, et al. Physician interpretations and textbook definitions of blinding terminology in randomized controlled trials. JAMA 2001; 285:2000–2003.
4. McGettigan P, Sly K, O'Connell D, et al. The effects of information framing on the practices of physicians. J Gen Intern Med 1999; 14:633–642.
5. Kristiansen IS, Gyrd-Hansen D, Nexoe J, et al. Number needed to treat: easily understood and intuitively meaningful? Theoretical considerations and a randomised trial. J Clin Epidemiol 2002; 55:888–892.
6. Torrance GW. Measurement of health state utilities for economic appraisal: a review. J Health Econ 1986; 5(1):1–30.
7. Sackett DL, Strauss SE, Richardson WS, et al. Evidence-Based Medicine. How to Practise and Teach EBM. 2nd edn. Edinburgh: Churchill Livingstone; 2000.
8. Moher D, Schulz KF, Altman DG. The consort statement: revised recommendations for improving the quality of reports of parallel group randomized trials. BMC Med Res Methodol 2001; 1:2.

5

Systematic reviews and meta-analysis

How do you summarize more than one study? In a traditional narrative review, the author, usually an expert, uses his or her knowledge to identify, appraise, and synthesize the literature to arrive at some conclusions. The methods used are not always the same and often unclear. Rarely do they use quantitative methods to combine the results of the studies. The methods used are idiosyncratic and implicit. In contrast, a systematic review uses explicit methods to systematically search, critically appraise, and synthesize the literature on a specific issue. For the reader who wishes to learn more about systematic reviews, we recommend the introductory texts by Mulrow and Cook[1] or Galsziou et al.[2] For those who wish to undertake systematic reviews themselves there are several advanced texts on the subject.[3,4,5]

Meta-analysis is the term used for the statistical procedures used to combine the results of several studies into a single pooled or summary estimate.[6] Although the terms systematic review and meta-analysis are sometimes used interchangeably, they refer to different types of summaries. You can have a systematic review that does not include a meta-analysis. For instance, the identified studies might be too different in goals or design, or similar outcome measures might not be able to be extracted, so that the results of studies might not able to be combined. It is also possible to have a meta-analysis of a set of studies which have not been systematically selected or appraised.

Both narrative and systematic reviews are retrospective, observational studies and are vulnerable to both bias and random error.[7] The quality of the review will depend on its methodological rigor, that is, the degree to which scientific review methods have been used to reduce bias and error. Table 5.1 contrasts narrative and systematic reviews. Narrative reviews are useful for:

- Describing the history or development of a problem;
- Describing new developments when the body of evidence is very limited or the studies are flawed;
- Discussing data in relation to theory; and
- Integrating different fields of research.

Table 5.1 Differences between narrative and systematic reviews (based Cook et al[7] with permission from American College of Physicians)

Feature	Narrative review	Systematic review
Question	Often broad in scope	Often a focused clinical question
Sources and search	Not usually specified, potentially biased	Comprehensive sources and explicit search strategy
Selection	Not usually specified, potentially biased	Criterion-based selection, uniformly applied
Appraisal	Variable	Rigorous critical appraisal
Synthesis	Often a qualitative summary	Usually a quantitative summary (meta-analysis)
Inferences	Sometimes evidence-based	Usually evidence-based

However, narrative reviews are more likely to be biased and provide imprecise estimates of effects compared to systematic reviews. They are also less likely to be contemporaneous with research and consequently make recommendations about treatment, which may be up to 10 years behind the research evidence.[8]

Rationale, advantages, and disadvantages

What is the rationale for systematic reviews? Information overload is a major problem for most clinicians, health care managers, funders and consumers of health care services. There are in excess of 20 000 health care journals and it is estimated that over 2 million articles are published each year. Many clinicians rely on summaries of current evidence to keep up-to-date, and systematic reviews can provide valid and accurate summaries of evidence in specific fields. There are also limited resources available to health researchers, and it is important that research effort is targeted towards gaps in the body of knowledge. Systematic reviews are a useful method for identifying such knowledge gaps. Additionally, health policy should be based on sound evidence, and systematic reviews can be used to inform the decisions of health policy makers.

There are some methodological advantages and disadvantages of systematic reviews.

- Many studies in psychiatry and psychology have limited statistical power and consequently are unable to detect small or modest effects.[9–12] By using meta-analytic procedures it is possible to aggregate the results of these studies and increase the power to demonstrate small or modest effects. However, the increased power is potentially a disadvantage as it allows the detection of small biases as well as small effects. This can result in a misleading estimate of the overall effect.

- By considering the effects across studies which differ in terms of setting, participants, mode of intervention, and other design features, it is possible to determine if the results are robust to these variations and generalizable. If the results of studies differ more than expected by chance (i.e. the studies are heterogeneous), then is possible to search for explanations for the variation.

Methodology of systematic review

A systematic review, like any scientific study, consists of a question (or hypothesis), a structured process (study design and analyses) that addresses the question, and a conclusion. The researcher attempts to make the processes explicit and takes steps to minimize bias (systematic error) and increase the precision (accuracy) of the findings. By making the processes explicit, the researcher deliberately opens the conduct of the study to external scrutiny and challenge. The processes should be sufficiently explicit to enable another researcher to repeat the study and determine whether the same results are achieved; if the findings are reproducible, they may be regarded as reliable. If the review is undertaken with appropriate rigor, the findings are also more likely to be valid (i.e. 'true'). Appendix 3 outlines the major steps in undertaking a review.

As discussed in Chapter 2, it is essential to have a clear question to be answered. The question should define: the group of persons with the disorder of interest (the 'target population'); the treatment, prognostic factor, etiological factor, or diagnostic test of interest (the 'intervention'); the group of persons who do not have the intervention and are used as a comparison (the 'comparison group'); and, the 'outcome' of interest (PICO). A well-framed question is the basis for an efficient literature search strategy and a rigorous review.

Finding studies (conduct literature search)

The validity of a systematic review is in part determined by whether all relevant studies (both published and unpublished) are identified. A comprehensive literature review will include most of the following elements:[13]

- Searches of major relevant electronic databases (Medline, EMBASE, Psychlit, the Cochrane Library);
- Handsearches of specific journals;
- Scanning of the bibliographies of the identified published studies;
- Using citation indexes to identify new studies that have cited key references;
- Handsearches of conference proceedings;
- Writing to active researchers and authors to ask if they can identify any unpublished studies and provide the data from such studies;
- Writing to industry (for instance, pharmaceutical companies) to ask if they can identify any unpublished studies and provide the data from such studies; and

- Writing to relevant government departments and international organizations to ask if they can identify any unpublished studies and provide the data from such studies.

Reliance on electronic databases alone, as a source of studies, will lead to incomplete identification of published studies.[14] Thus, a comprehensive search strategy will include handsearches of relevant journals, scanning of bibliographies, and searching with citation indexes. Most electronic databases will not include unpublished studies, the exception to this being the Cochrane Library. Therefore, it is important to attempt to identify the unpublished studies by searching conference proceedings and directly contacting individuals or organizations likely to have knowledge of and access to the results of unpublished studies.

Apply inclusion and exclusion criteria

Before undertaking the search for studies, the researchers should define explicit criteria for the inclusion or exclusion of studies in the systematic review. The inclusion and exclusion criteria may be based on:

- The study participants;
- The disorder or problem of interest;
- The design and conduct of the study; on
- The outcomes of interest.

The researcher will use these predefined criteria, to develop checklists, which may be used to determine which studies should be included or excluded. It is good practice to have two or more researchers independently review the identified studies to determine whether the studies meet the inclusion criteria. When the reviewers disagree about whether a particular study should be included, they will meet to discuss the issues and arrive at a consensus decision. It is also good practice that the reviewers be blind to the authors' names, the authors' institutions, and the publication details (i.e. journal, year of publication, country of publication). These latter measures (independent reviewers, blinding of reviewers) minimize the likelihood that the reviewers will be consciously or unconsciously influenced in their decision making by factors other than the inclusion and exclusion criteria. In the systematic review, the researchers should provide tables of the included and excluded studies with a brief explanation of the reasons for exclusion of studies.

Data abstraction

The researchers should determine what data they wish to document from the included studies and develop forms to record the abstracted data. It is wise to pilot these forms, and modify them if required, before beginning the data extraction proper. As with the inclusion–exclusion of studies, it is preferred that the data abstraction is undertaken independently by two or more persons, with any differences in the data extracted investigated and resolved by consensus. Again, it is preferable that the data abstraction be undertaken blind to the authors' names, the authors' institutions, and the publication details (i.e. journal, year of publication, country of publication). In the write-up of the review, the authors should briefly describe what data was abstracted and the procedures they used.

Conduct analysis

As with any scientific study, the reviewers should have an analysis plan that specifies the types of analyses which will be undertaken and how the results will be presented. As with many areas of research, meta-analysis has become an area of specialization for biostatisticians. Although there are a number of packages, which greatly ease the conduct of meta-analysis, the appropriate application of meta-analytic techniques and the interpretation of results requires training and expertise. The research team should include a biostatistician or have access to a biostatistician who has expertise in this area.

Determining the applicability of results

In the final part of a systematic review (usually in the 'Discussion' section), the reviewers must consider how the results might be interpreted and applied to relevant clinical populations. The reviewers should consider how similar or dissimilar the participants in the studies are to the patient populations of interest. The participant characteristics that might be considered include age, gender, socioeconomic standing, illness severity, diagnosis, and the presence of co-morbid conditions. The reviewers should also consider the mode of delivery of the intervention of interest in the studies: how similar was the treatment to that used in usual clinical settings? Finally, the reviewers should consider the outcomes measured in the studies and whether such outcomes are meaningful, both in terms of the outcome type and size of the effect on outcomes, to clinicians, and patients.

Meta-analysis

As discussed earlier, meta-analytic procedures are specialist statistical procedures that require knowledge and expertise to be used and interpreted appropriately. Although statistical software has made such procedures more accessible to researchers, this has increased the likelihood that a naive researcher will misuse or misinterpret the results of tests. In this section, we will provide a brief outline of the major elements of meta-analysis for systematic reviews, but for more detail and a presentation of the theoretical basis of the procedures, the reader should consult a specialist text such as Sutton et al.[4] or the relevant chapters in Egger et al.[3]

Data synthesis

If there are a sufficient number of excluded studies, from which a measure of effect and variation can be extracted, and these studies are sufficiently similar ('homogeneous'), then it is possible to combine the results from the studies and obtain an estimate of the overall effect and an estimate of the overall variation. Usually the results are combined by taking a weighted average of the individual study results, most often according to sample size.[15] The results of the studies can be combined using statistical procedures based on two different models: the fixed effects and the random effects models.

With the fixed effects model, it is assumed that there is one 'true' underlying population value, of which the individual studies provide estimates. The random effects model assumes there are a number of population values, of which the individual studies provide a random sample of estimates. The random effects model takes into account both within- and between-study variation when calculating an overall estimation of variation. Although there is not a 'correct' model, it is advisable to use the random effects model when there is significant between-study variation (i.e. heterogeneity).

Effect sizes

The method by which effect estimates from different studies are combined will vary depending on the type of outcome measures. There are two classes of measure: those associated with dichotomous measures (e.g. death/survival, recovery/nonrecovery), and those associated with continuous measures (e.g. improvement as measured with the Hamilton Depression Scale). Table 5.2 below lists some commonly used outcome measures with definitions.

By convention, outcome measures are usually calculated with respect to adverse outcomes, for instance, death, or the occurrence of some adverse event. In studies in psychiatry and other areas of mental health, it is more usual to measure positive outcomes, such as recovery or symptom reduction. It is possible to use the same measures and formulae to calculate the outcome measures for positive benefits.

Heterogeneity

In a systematic review and in meta-analysis, it is important to search for possible sources of variation, or 'heterogeneity', between the studies, especially when the estimates of effect are significantly different.

Table 5.2 Commonly used measures of outcome and their definitions (adapted from, Glasziou et al[2], with permission from Cambridge University Press)

Outcome measure	Definition
Odds ratio	Ratio of the odds of the outcome in the intervention group to the odds in the comparison group
Relative risk	The ratio of the risk of the outcome (or proportion with the outcome) in the intervention group to the risk of the outcome (or proportion with the outcome) in the comparison group
Absolute risk difference	The difference between the proportion in the intervention group with the outcome and the proportion in the comparison group
Number-needed-to-treat	The number of patients who have to be treated to avoid one adverse event. It can be calculated as the reciprocal of the absolute risk difference
Weighted difference in means	The average difference between the intervention and control groups in the estimates of the means of the outcomes from all the included studies. The outcome measurement is in the same natural scale for all included studies
Standardized weighted mean difference	The average standardized difference between the intervention and control groups in the estimates of the means of the outcomes from all the included studies. This is used when the outcome measurement is in different scales for the included studies (for instance, different anxiety measurement scales)

Heterogeneity may be the result of actual or apparent differences among the studies. Examples of sources of actual differences may include:

- Differences in the timing of measurement of the outcome-of-interest;
- Differences in the severity of disorder in the studies' participants, or the presence of co-morbid conditions;
- Differences in intensity, duration, or timing of the intervention; and
- The presence of additional treatments.

Sources of apparent differences in outcomes may include:

- Inaccurate measurement of outcome;
- Poor adherence with treatment by the participants; and
- Poor study design such as poor concealment of allocation (i.e. faulty randomization) or poor blinding of assessors of outcome.

There are a number of statistical tests used to assess heterogeneity. A commonly used test is the Cochrane chi-square (or 'Cochrane Q' test), which may be simply interpreted as indicating the presence of heterogeneity when the p-value is significant. A range of other tests and procedures are available, and the interested reader should consult more detailed texts for more information. If a meta-analysis shows that results are consistent across studies despite real differences between studies, this would suggest that the estimate of the treatment effect and variation are robust. That is, it is reasonable to generalize the results to a range of patient populations and clinical contexts. If real differences are found and these predict the size of treatment effect, then the sources of these real differences may be important to the understanding of the disorder or treatment response.

Publication bias

Publication bias is defined as '(the) type of bias which arises due to selective publication in medical journals of results which report statistically significant results'. It is with the intent of avoiding publication bias that vigorous efforts are made in the literature search to identify all relevant studies, both published and unpublished. However, it is still possible that, despite the best efforts of the reviewers, publication bias may be present. The reviewers should look for this possibility.

It is possible to look for publication bias using a simple graph known as a 'funnel plot' (Fig. 5.1). With a funnel plot, the sizes of the treatment effects (from the individual studies) are plotted against the reciprocals of the standard errors (a measure of precision). Studies with smaller numbers of participants are likely to be underpowered to demonstrate a true difference among the groups, when a true difference is present. Such studies with negative findings are also less likely to be published if publication bias is present. This pattern will be evident on the funnel plot as gaps in the tails of the funnel.

There are also a number of statistical tests which may be used to detect publication bias. These include the Rank Correlation Test (also known as the Begg and Mazumbar test) and the Linear Regression Test (also known as Egger's test). More information on these tests is provided

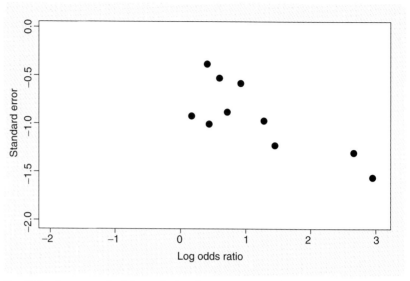

Fig. 5.1 Asymmetrical funnel plot (*http://www.cochrane-net.org/openlearning/HTML/mod15-3.htm* Copyright Cochrane Library, reproduced with permission).

in Chapter 7 of Sutton et al.[4] If publication bias is present, the reviewers may make further attempts to locate missing trials or may adjust the results of the meta-analysis using statistical techniques. However, the evidence supporting the latter techniques is poor and such approaches should be used and interpreted with caution.

Subgroup analysis

From some studies it may be possible to abstract data on the outcomes for subgroups of participants. Such subgroups may be defined on the basis of participant characteristics (age, gender) or disorder characteristics (severity, duration, symptom type). Reviewers may choose to assess the size of treatment effects in these subgroups, or make comparisons with other subgroups. Such subgroup analyses are often inappropriate because of the inadequate sample sizes or the fact that multiple significance testing will increase the likelihood of a statistically significant difference appearing by chance. Because of the latter possibility, it is preferable that subgroup testing be undertaken on an *a priori* basis. Subgroup analysis is best regarded as an exploratory technique, which may show interesting differences that will require confirmation in further studies.

Sensitivity analysis

Sensitivity analysis is a strategy which allows interviewers to explore how robust their findings are to the assumptions that underpin the systematic review and meta-analysis. Essentially, the reviewers repeat the analyses while changing an assumption to see if this changes the findings. An example would be to change the inclusion/exclusion criteria for studies and see if this leads to different findings. This might include the inclusion/exclusion of published/unpublished studies or the inclusion/exclusion of studies of poorer methodological quality. Similarly, the statistical model used (fixed effects or random effects) might be changed to see if this is associated with a change in findings. If the review findings are sensitive to changes in underlying assumptions, then the findings might be interpreted with caution.

Data presentation

It is usual to present the results of meta-analyses in tabular and graphical forms that ease the assimilation and interpretation of the information for the reader. The standard form of graphical presentation is the 'forest plot' (Fig. 5.2). In a forest plot each individual study is presented as point

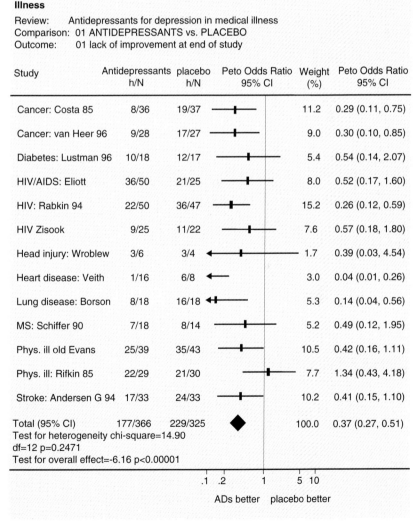

Illness

Review: Antidepressants for depression in medical illness
Comparison: 01 ANTIDEPRESSANTS vs. PLACEBO
Outcome: 01 lack of improvement at end of study

Study	Antidepressants h/N	placebo h/N	Peto Odds Ratio 95% CI	Weight (%)	Peto Odds Ratio 95% CI
Cancer: Costa 85	8/36	19/37		11.2	0.29 (0.11, 0.75)
Cancer: van Heer 96	9/28	17/27		9.0	0.30 (0.10, 0.85)
Diabetes: Lustman 96	10/18	12/17		5.4	0.54 (0.14, 2.07)
HIV/AIDS: Eliott	36/50	21/25		8.0	0.52 (0.17, 1.60)
HIV: Rabkin 94	22/50	36/47		15.2	0.26 (0.12, 0.59)
HIV Zisook	9/25	11/22		7.6	0.57 (0.18, 1.80)
Head injury: Wroblew	3/6	3/4		1.7	0.39 (0.03, 4.54)
Heart disease: Veith	1/16	6/8		3.0	0.04 (0.01, 0.26)
Lung disease: Borson	8/18	16/18		5.3	0.14 (0.04, 0.56)
MS: Schiffer 90	7/18	8/14		5.2	0.49 (0.12, 1.95)
Phys. ill old Evans	25/39	35/43		10.5	0.42 (0.16, 1.11)
Phys. ill: Rifkin 85	22/29	21/30		7.7	1.34 (0.43, 4.18)
Stroke: Andersen G 94	17/33	24/33		10.2	0.41 (0.15, 1.10)
Total (95% CI)	177/366	229/325		100.0	0.37 (0.27, 0.51)

Test for heterogeneity chi-square=14.90
df=12 p=0.2471
Test for overall effect=-6.16 p<0.00001

.1 .2   1   5 10

ADs better   placebo better

Fig. 5.2 'Forest plot' for a systematic review of antidepressants in physical illness.

and line. The size of the point is proportional either to the number of participants in the study or the precision of the study (the reciprocal of the standard error). The line represents the confidence intervals – usually the 95% confidence intervals of the estimates. The studies may be organized on the graph in chronological order or by width of confidence intervals. If an overall estimate of effect size and variance has been calculated, this is usually represented as a diamond at the bottom of the graph. The width of the diamond represents the confidence intervals and the area of the diamond is proportional to either the total number of participants or the precision of the estimate. To one side of the graph and alongside the appropriate graphical representation of each individual study, it is usual to present the total number of participants in each arm of the study. When the outcome is dichotomous, the number in each arm who had the outcome of interest will also be included. For odds ratios and relative risk, a vertical line is drawn up from 1.0, which is the point of no difference. If the confidence interval crosses this line, the finding is not significant. If the confidence interval does not cross the line, the study shows either a significant benefit or disadvantage for the intervention group. By convention, it is usual to show a beneficial effect with points to the left of the line (i.e. rations of less than 1.0).

An initiative to improve the quality of reporting of meta-analyses of randomized controlled trials is the QUORUM statement.[16]

Users' guides for how to use review articles

With this background, the reader is now in a position to critically appraise a systematic review. The questions in Box 5.1 are obtained from the JAMA series of papers titled 'Users' Guides to the Medical Literature'; these guides have been updated and collected together in a text edited by Guyatt and Rennie.[17] Similar guides may be found in Sackett et al.[5]

The Cochrane Collaboration

The Cochrane Collaboration is an international organization which has as its primary purpose the production and dissemination of high-quality systematic reviews of randomized controlled trials of interventions, in all areas of health care. These reviews are regularly updated to ensure they are current. The collaboration provides training and technical support for persons who wish to undertake reviews. Although the terms Cochrane review and systematic review have almost become synonymous, it is important to note that not all systematic reviews are Cochrane reviews. Furthermore, although the Cochrane Collaboration has chosen to focus on reviews of randomized controlled trials, it is possible to undertake reviews of other types of studies including studies of prevalence, diagnostic tests, etiology and prognosis.[2]

Box 5.1   Appraisal of a systematic review

Are the results valid?

- Did the review explicitly address a sensible clinical question?
- Was the search for relevant studies detailed and exhaustive?
- Were the primary studies of high methodological quality?
- Were assessments of studies reproducible?

What are the results?

- Were the results similar from study to study?
- What are the overall results of the review?
- How precise were the results?

How can I apply the results to patient care?

- How can I best interpret the results to apply them to the care of the patients in my practice?
- Were all the clinically important outcomes considered?
- Are the benefits worth the costs and potential risks?

Summary

A systematic review is useful for identifying and summarizing the information from studies in a particular field. However, the conduct of a systematic review is time consuming; the meta-analysis is fraught with hazard unless undertaken with care and expert guidance. Despite the difficulties, the number of systematic reviews published annually is increasing rapidly. Systematic reviews are often used in the development of decision-support tools such as clinical practice guidelines and decision analyses. It is important that clinicians, administrators, funders, providers, and policy analysts in mental health be familiar with the methodology of systematic reviews and be able to critically appraise such reviews.

References

1. Mulrow CD, Cook D, eds. Systematic Reviews. Synthesis of Best Evidence for Health Care Decisions. 1st ed. Philadelphia: American College of Physicians; 1998.
2. Glasziou P, et al. Systematic Reviews in Health Care. A Practical Guide. 1st edn. Cambridge: Cambridge University Press; 2001.
3. Egger M, Davey Smith G, Altman DG eds. Systematic Reviews in Health Care. Meta-analysis in Context. 2nd edn. London: BMJ Publishing Group; 2001.
4. Sutton AJ, et al. Methods for Meta-analysis in Medical Research. 1st edn. Wiley Series in Probability and Statistics. Chichester: John Wiley & Sons Ltd; 2000.
5. Sackett DL, et al. Evidence-based Medicine. How to Practise and Teach EBM. 2nd edn. Edinburgh: Churchill Livingstone; 2000.
6. Oxman A, et al. Summarizing the Evidence, in: Users' Guides to the Medical Literature. Essentials of Evidence-Based Clinical Practice. Guyatt G, Rennie D, Eds. Chicago: American Medical Association; 2002; p. 241–269.
7. Cook DJ, Mulrow CD, Haynes RB. Synthesis of Best Evidence for Clinical Decisions in: Systematic Reviews. Synthesis of Best Evidence for Health Care Decisions. Mulrow CD, Cook D, eds. Philadelphia: American College of Physicians; 1998: pp. 5–12.

8. Antman EM, et al. A comparison of results of meta-analyses of randomized control trials and recommendations of clinical experts. Treatments for myocardial infarction. JAMA 1992; 268:240–248.

9. Bird KD, Hall W. Statistical power in psychiatric research. Aust N Z J Psychiatry 1986; 20(2):189–200.

10. Cohen J. The statistical power of abnormal social psychological research: a review. J Abnorm Soc Psychol 1962; 65:145–153.

11. Rossi JS. Statistical power of psychological research: what have we gained in 20 years? J Consult Clin Psychol 1990; 58:646–656.

12. Kazdin AE, Bass D. Power to detect differences between alternative treatments in comparative psychotherapy outcome research. J Consul Clin Psychol 1989; 57: 138–147.

13. McKibbon A, Eady A, Marks S. Chapter 6: Secondary publications: systematic review articles, in: PDQ evidence-based Principles and Practice. McKibbon A, Eady A, Marks S. eds. Hamilton: BC Decker Inc.; 1999: pp. 121–151.

14. Adams CE, et al. An investigation of the adequacy of MEDLINE searches for randomized controlled trials (RCTs) of the effects of mental health care. Psycholog Med 1994; 24:741–748.

15. Pereira-Maxwell F. A–Z of Medical Statistics. London; Arnold Publishers: 1998.

16. Moher D, Cook DJ, Eastwood S, et al. Improving the quality of reports of meta-analyses of randomized controlled trials: the QUORUM statement. Quality of reporting of meta-analyses. Lancet 1999; 354: 1896–1900.

17. Guyatt G, Rennie D, eds. Users' Guides to the Medical Literature. Essentials of Evidence-Based Practice. 1st edn. Chicago: American Medical Association; 2002.

6

Putting evidence to use – clinical practice guidelines

What are clinical practice guidelines?

Clinical practice guidelines are statements that have been written to help professionals deliver good health care. Good guidelines have been developed systematically and help decision making in clearly defined situations. The concept is not new and guidelines have been around for many years. An example of a well-established clinical practice guideline is a flow chart for managing cardiac arrests. During the few minutes following a cardiac arrest it is difficult to make carefully thought-out decisions about defibrillating or injecting drugs yourself and there is no time to turn to the literature! Cardiac arrest charts are widely accepted as helpful.

What has changed recently is the realization that clinical guidelines can be helpful in a wider range of complex clinical situations. It has also become clear that they should be evidence based. At first sight, it has been argued that mental health does not lend itself well to guidelines. Mental illness is not as clear-cut as ventricular fibrillation or asystole. Similarly, the treatments for mental illness are not as simple as defibrillation or adrenaline. However, there is growing evidence that guidelines can be helpful for complex situations for general and mental health.

Guidelines lend themselves well to evidence-based care because they are transparent. What a clinician says or does with a client in a consulting room is usually private. Some clinicians emphasize the importance of the sanctity of the one-to-one clinician–patient relationship and are reluctant to demystify it. Sometimes it is for good reasons – it is impossible to reduce the whole of an interaction between two individuals to a series of statements on a piece of paper. However, resistance can also come for bad reasons, such as an anxiety that the clinician will somehow lose power if the interaction becomes explicit.

What can clinical practice guidelines achieve?

Guidelines can provide recommendations for clinicians managing their patients' care. They can also be used to develop standards to assess the clinical practice of mental health professionals. They can be used for the education and training of clinicians as well as helping patients to make informed decisions. They can also be used to improve communication between professionals and patients.

Patients' own experiences

One criticism of evidence-based guidelines is that they do not leave room for a patient's individual experience because this is seen as subjective. However, evidence-based guidelines can benefit from individual experiences and from group experiences through studies such as case histories and qualitative designs. Room can be made for putting the guidelines into context, and this may include broader issues about service provisions and different viewpoints.

How do clinical practice guidelines differ from protocols and evidence-based summaries?

There are lots of different terms used for clinical practice guidelines. In particular, the term is often used interchangeably with protocol. However, protocols are usually defined as systems that are expected to be followed closely. The name suggests that guidelines are only guides and consequently do not have to be followed, whereas protocols are established practice and need to be carried out. In practice, clinicians may find some guidelines as important to follow as protocols and use the terms interchangeably.

Evidence-based guidelines are those that should have been developed after systematically appraising the literature, whereas consensus-based guidelines are at a lower level of evidence and rely on the consensus of a group of experts. The grade of evidence for each recommendation should always be recorded (Table 6.1). Evidence-based summaries are a condensing of available evidence but not a statement written to guide care.

Table 6.1   A hierarchy of evidence for treatment guidelines

Level	Type of evidence
Ia	A systematic review and meta-analysis of RCTs
Ib	At least one RCT
IIa	At least one well-designed controlled study
IIb	At least one well-designed quasi-experimental study
III	Well-designed nonexperimental studies, such as case studies or comparative studies
IV	Expert opinion

Clinical practice guidelines as a reaction to the variation in practice of health care

It has been widely recognized for some time that the management of mental illness can often be improved. There are many reasons for this, including the complexity of mental illness, the consequent poor understanding of it, and the poor resources and stigmatization it has traditionally received. These reasons also partly explain the huge variation in mental health care delivered across countries and parts of countries. Therefore, there have been attempts to drive up standards. One attempt is clinical audit and another clinical guidelines. These processes lend themselves to be used together.

What are the features of a good guideline?

A well-written clinical guideline will offer clear recommendations that are usable and flexible. The process of their development will be transparent and include the involvement of all parties affected by its use. The recommendations will be evidence based and the grade of available evidence will be included. The results should be both reliable and valid. A time-scale will show over what period the literature was searched and when it should be reviewed. Thought will have been applied to how to implement the guideline and this will be explicit.

Where to find clinical practice guidelines

There are a number of ways of finding clinical guidelines. A number of organizations have taken on the roles of developing, coordinating, or collecting guidelines. They also offer help in developing guidelines and useful tools, such as a tools for evaluating and comparing guidelines. Some of the main organizations are listed in Table 6.2. They can be found on the Internet and have search engines for protocols. A further source is searching archives such as Medline, as outlined in the previous chapter. A search at the National Guideline Clearinghouse (NGC) website for guidelines about depression retrieves well over 150 matches.

The process of creating a guideline

Traditionally, guidelines have been based on a consensus among experts. However, this process is often flawed. Experts may not be aware of the latest evidence and if they are, may not have appraised it. Experts may be overly influenced by their own practice, where individual successes could be weighed too heavily even though they may have arisen by chance. Experts may be more experienced with unusual cases that have been referred to specialist centers and not the more common presentations. There have been many interventions in mental health

Table 6.2 Sources for guidelines

Organization	Website	Country	Description
National Guideline Clearinghouse (NGC)	*www.guideline.gov*	USA	Offers a comprehensive database of evidence-based clinical practice guidelines
The National Institute of Clinical Evidence (NICE)	*www.nice.org.uk*	UK	Produces guidelines at the request of the United Kingdom Department of Health
The New Zealand Guidelines Group (NZGG)	*www.nzgg.org.nz*	New Zealand	Promotes effective delivery of health and disability services, based on evidence

endorsed by experts but later found to be ineffective or with risks that outweigh benefits (for example insulin coma therapy). Developers of a guideline need to be aware of their own possible biases. The guidelines should rely on the best possible evidence available, and only in the absence of good evidence be based on expert judgment through consensus statements.

The process for developing guidelines should be inclusive and systematic (Box 6.1). Developing evidence-based guidelines is time consuming and expensive and usually undertaken in consultation with organizations such as those listed above.

Developing a guideline
Identifying an area

The first step is to identify an area that may benefit from a guideline. The primary aim will be to improve health. Could a guideline reduce illness, disability, or deaths? Can a guideline improve efficiency and save money to spend on other interventions? Will it contribute to an area

---

Box 6.1 Principles underlying guideline development at the National Institute of Clinical Evidence

Clinical guidelines should:

Aim to improve the quality of clinical care.

Address clinical effectiveness.

Address cost effectiveness.

Be advisory.

Be developed through a process that considers all those who may be affected by the guideline.

Be based on the best possible research evidence and professional consensus.

Be developed using principles that command respect of patients and other groups.

Be developed with the involvement of patients and health care professionals.

considered a priority by local or national bodies? Will it help reduce variations in clinical care? There are already a large number of guidelines for assessing and managing mental health problems. Some may not have been developed with an evidence base and can be improved; others may be poorly constructed or out of date. The more specific the guideline, the easier it will be to develop. For example, a guideline for managing mental health problems would be too broad to be practicable. A guideline for managing anxiety disorder is more specific and achievable. You need to identify the settings and the professional groups. For a guideline for managing schizophrenia, is it in primary health care for GPs or is it for managing inpatients by nurses? Discuss the topic with colleagues and relevant organizations to see if they feel a guideline may be helpful.

Defining the question

The principals of defining guideline questions are similar to those discussed in the chapter on formulating answerable questions. It can be helpful to use the **PICO** system – **P**atient or population of interest; **I**ntervention; **C**omparison; **O**utcome. For example, if you were thinking of developing a clinical practice guideline for using mechanical restraints in a mental health unit, you could start by formulating a question as below (Table 6.3).

Having the correct aims

It is important at an early stage to identify why you are developing a guideline. The principal aim should be to improve the quality of clinical care. Other aims may be to improve efficiency, standardise care, and improve communication with patients.

Estimating the cost

It is good practice to include an analysis of the cost implications of a guideline (Box 6.2). There is a finite amount of money available to spend on mental health care, and almost all services struggle with sub-optimal funding. Under these conditions, priorities need to be set and this process is made easier by having transparent costs for managing different conditions and situations. Some agencies may be more keen to implement a clinical practice guideline if it is shown to come with a cost benefit as well as a clinical benefit. There are a number of different ways of costing a guideline. The first step will be to search the literature for existing economic analyses. If these are inadequate, a cost-impact assessment should be undertaken and this may involve developing models to

Table 6.3 A clinical practice guideline (therapy) question

The **Patient**	For an acutely disturbed patient on a mental health unit
The **Intervention**	Using mechanical restraints
The **Comparison** if relevant	Not using restraints
The **Outcome**	Improves patient and staff safety

Box 6.2   Competing interests and developing guidelines

There are concerns that most guidelines on clinical practice are written by experts with undisclosed links to the pharmaceutical industry.[1] In a survey of nearly 200 authors of 44 clinical guidelines, 87% of respondents admitted to financial links with one or more pharmaceutical company.[2] Over half of the authors had been paid to conduct research, over a third had been an employee or a consultant, and two-thirds had received fees for speaking. On average, each respondent had links with 10 companies, including companies whose products they recommended in guidelines. Only one of the 44 guidelines carried a declaration of the authors' competing interests. Most (93%) of the respondents said their relationship with the pharmaceutical companies did not affect their recommendations on treatment. The researchers were unable to check whether authors' financial links did influence the guidelines because there were too few independent guidelines to make a meaningful comparison. The researchers called for a formal process to be built into guideline development that forces authors to declare their financial interests. They also wanted written declarations of competing interests on every guideline.

---

come to the best estimates. The development group should include a health economist who can help explore the costs of various interventions.

Local guideline or national guideline

You need to be clear whether you are developing a local guideline for use in your own service or a guideline aimed at wider usage. Local guidelines are usually easier to develop and have the advantage of involving the professionals who will implement the guideline from the start. National guidelines might already be available and can be adapted for local use.

Involving the right people

The next step is to involve a number of key individuals and organizations in drawing up the guidelines. These people should include representatives from the health professions involved in delivering the care and patient groups for whom the guidelines are written. Guidelines are more likely to be used by professionals if they have some ownership of them (Box 6.3). Guidelines developed by senior members of an organization and disseminated downwards may be used reluctantly or not at all. There may also be a tension between a 'management' perspective of delivering care within certain resources and a 'clinician' perspective of delivering the best care to the individual patient.

Finding the evidence base

The next step is to examine the evidence base for the clinical situation. The steps for this are discussed in other chapters and include a thorough search of the literature for different grades of evidence (Table 6.4).

Writing the guideline

You should identify what the grade of evidence is for each step. Each step of the process needs to be recorded so the whole development process of the guideline is transparent.

> **Box 6.3**   A controversial guideline
>
> The *BMJ* reported the media furor that erupted even before clinical practice guidelines for chronic fatigue syndrome were published in Australia.[3] 'Sick and tired patients in uproar', blared one front page headline of a leading daily newspaper. The chairman of the ME/CFS Association of Australia, Simon Molesworth, was quoted as saying that the guidelines trivialized the condition, blamed sufferers, and would encourage misdiagnosis, inappropriate medical care, and misconceptions about the illness. Craig Ellis, the Consumers' Health Forum representative on the guidelines committee, who consulted widely with other people with CFS during the six years of the guidelines process, agreed with their publication and said that the committee had mostly accommodated consumer concerns about earlier drafts. The controversy settled somewhat when Mr Molesworth and Professor Larkins, president of the Royal Australasian College of Physicians, who developed the guidelines, agreed on certain areas. However, the furor did raise the wider issue of divergent views that can exist between professionals and consumer groups. Consumers can feel frustrated that the evidence-based process of guideline development leaves little room for inclusion of their personal experiences.

Testing the guideline

Before it is implemented, it can be tried by professionals not involved in the writing to look at it for consistency and clarity. You need to arrange a randomized controlled trial to see if the guideline actually improves care.

Reviewing the guideline

A guideline will need to be regularly reviewed to take into account new knowledge. Time-frames are useful, such as identifying that the guideline will need to be reviewed in 12 months. New developments in mental health care may mean the guideline has to be reviewed sooner than anticipated.

Disseminating the guideline

The guideline needs to be publicized to the relevant professionals. This should be done in a variety of ways, including meetings, conferences, road shows, educational programs, and the Internet.

Implementing the guideline

This is the more active process of ensuring that the relevant professionals are using the guideline. Structural changes (e.g. workload and resources) need to be considered as well as attitudinal changes (e.g. professionals' willingness to change behaviour).

Table 6.4   Typical grading of recommendations[4]

Grade	Evidence
A	At least one RCT as part of a body of literature of overall good quality and consistency addressing the specific recommendation (evidence levels Ia and Ib)
B	Well-conducted clinical studies but no RCTs on the topic of the recommendation (evidence levels IIa, IIb, III)
C	Expert committee reports or opinions and/or clinical experience of respected authorities. The grading indicates that directly applicable clinical studies of good quality are absent (evidence level IV)

Auditing the guideline

Using clinical audit can improve the use of a guideline. The audit cycle is a process in which an assessment is made as to how often the various parts of the guideline are being used. These results are presented to the professionals involved, and implementation processes are reconsidered and implemented. Then the audit is repeated to see if there is any change. Audit can be used as a continuous process to improve the use of the guideline.

What to include in a guideline

A guideline will include the central recommendations and the grade of evidence supporting those recommendations. However, a number of other details will help others understand how the guideline was developed and its scope. The profile of interventions assessed by the development should be included as well as a description of how the evidence was collected, reviewed, and assessed. There will be a full list of references to the literature and details of those who were involved in developing the guideline or who were consulted. Advice may be included about implementation and some time-frames included for review.

Versions of a clinical practice guideline

There may be more than one version of the guideline. A shortened version should make access to the key recommendations easier. It could include a clinical practice algorithm. This is a flow chart presented on one page that summarizes the steps in the guideline. It makes reference to longer versions of the guideline where necessary. A full guideline version will include all the information detailed above. A patient version of the guideline often interprets the recommendations in a shortened form for patients and carers. The aim will be to help patients make informed decisions about their care. It can be made available for patient or carer organizations to reproduce in their own literature.

Clinical algorithms

It is often helpful to include a clinical algorithm with the clinical practice guideline. This is diagrammatic representation of the steps taken to follow the recommendations of the guideline (Fig. 6.1). An algorithm is usually written to fill one page so it can be easily referred to. More details and references for each of the steps are included in the main guideline. Different aspects of care of the same condition can be included in one algorithm such as acute presentations, longer standing illness, treatment-resistant illness, or pathways to care.

An example of an evidence-based clinical guideline

One example is a guideline for assessing and treating anxiety disorders on the New Zealand Guidelines Group website (Box 6.4). The first section explains the purpose of the guideline and who it is aimed at. The guideline team had 15 members from several disciplines and included two consumer representatives. Conflicts of interests are not listed. The summary, designed for busy health care workers, includes brief information about anxiety and different approaches to identifying and

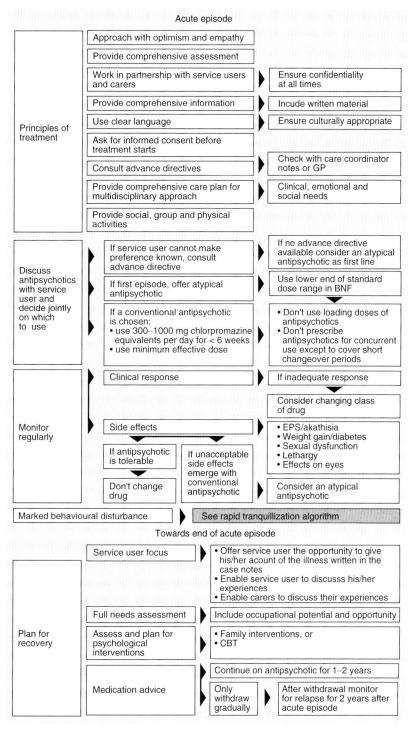

Fig. 6.1 An example of part of a clinical algorithm for treating schizophrenia, from the NHS National Institute for Clinical Excellence (*www.nice.org.uk*) Clinical Guideline No.12, with permission.

Box 6.4   New Zealand Guidelines Group: structure of guidelines for assessing and treating anxiety disorders

Contents

- Purpose of the Guideline
- About the Guideline
  - *Foreword from the National Health Committee*
  - *Guideline Team*
  - *Documentation*
- Guideline Information
  - *Summary*
  - *Table of Contents*
  - *Algorithms*
    - Differentiating Anxiety Disorders
    - Summary of Assessment and Initial Treatment
    - Treating Concurrent Anxiety and Substance Use
    - Treating Concurrent Anxiety and Depression
  - *Full Guideline*

---

managing anxiety disorders. There are four algorithms, each easily reducible to one side of A4 paper. The main report is 80 pages long and includes a lot of information about the anxiety disorders. Key recommendations come with a grading of the strength of evidence, although most are at the expert consensus level. There is no date for review.

Guidelines on guidelines

Reassuringly there are guidelines on guidelines! These are guides for appraising the quality of guidelines and are available from the websites described in Table 6.2. Like the critical appraisal questions elsewhere in this book, they boil down to questions of validity, importance, and relevance. The markers of quality (validity) are: did the authors of the guideline carry out a systematic search of the literature and were the recommendations in the guideline linked to a specific reference and a level of evidence? Indicators of relevance and importance are often blurred together. Sackett[5] describes the four B's as questions which indicate relevance and importance: What is the burden of illness in the local community? What are the beliefs of the community about the value of the interventions? What is the cost of implementation; is it a bad bargain? Are the barriers to carrying out the intervention too high to make it worth while?

Do guidelines make any difference to patient care?

There is evidence that guidelines can improve patient care. A review of 59 guideline evaluation studies found that in all but four statistically significant improvements occurred in clinical practice after implementation.[6] A systematic review of 87 studies on the use of guidelines concluded that 81 studies showed evidence of improved patient outcomes.[7] A systematic review of the effects of clinical practice guidelines in nursing, midwifery, and other health professionals allied to medicine found 18 studies.[8] They concluded there is some evidence that guideline-driven care is effective in changing processes and outcome. However, a review of quantitative studies of adherence to mental health clinical practice guidelines found that guideline adherence is not high without specific intervention.[9] Successful interventions tended to be complex, involving system redesign or additional resources.

The importance of dissemination and implementation

As much effort needs to go into the dissemination and implementation of a guideline as developing the guideline itself. Clinicians are more likely to use a guideline if they have some ownership of it and perceive it as useful. There is likely to be resistance if it is seen as imposed, bureaucratic, or irrelevant. Consumers are more likely to see it as useful if consumers were involved in the process and their concerns addressed.

References

1. Tonks A. Authors of guidelines have strong links with drugs industry. News. BMJ 2002; 324:383.
2. Choudhry NK, Stelfox HT, Detsky AS. Relationships between authors of clinical practice guidelines and the pharmaceutical industry. JAMA 2002; 287:612–617.
3. Sweet M. Chronic fatigue syndrome guidelines spark media row. News. BMJ 2002; 324:1284.
4. National Institute of Clinical Evidence. The guideline development process Series No 1. *www.nice.org.uk.*
5. Sackett DL, Strauss SE, Richardson WS, et al. Evidence-Based Medicine. How to Practise and Teach EBM. 2nd edn. Edinburgh: Churchill Livingstone; 2000.
6. Grimshaw J, Russell I. Effects of clinical guidelines on medical practice: a systematic review of rigorous evaluations. Lancet 1993; 342:1317–1322.
7. Effective Health Care Bulletin. Implementing clinical practice guidelines. York: University of York; 1994.
8. Thomas L, Cullum N, McColl E, Rousseau N, Soutter J, Steen N. Guidelines in professions allied to medicine (Cochrane Review). In: The Cochrane Library, 2004, Issue 2. Chichester: John Wiley; 2004.
9. Bauer MS. A review of quantitative studies of adherence to mental health clinical practice guidelines. Harv Rev Psychiatry 2002; 10:138–153.

7

What is the cause?

The theory of cause

There are few areas of health care where cause A can be said to cause outcome B. Even in the field of infectious diseases, for example, it is not sufficient to say that the tubercle bacillus causes tuberculosis. The individuals who get TB have been exposed to TB but there is nearly always something else, for example poor nutrition, to make them susceptible to becoming infected. What we are normally left with in studies of cause, whatever the study method, is a statement that an exposure increases the probability of developing a disorder. The problem is explaining why the exposure does not always cause the disorder. The solution appears to be to think about multifactorial causes 'acting together like musical instruments in an orchestra' rather than randomly and independently. Causes act conditionally upon other causes being present, and in combination they become sufficient to cause the disorder. There may also be several different groupings of factors that result in a disorder.[1] This way of thinking helps to frame questions about cause. Instead of 'Does A cause B?' the question becomes 'What role does A have in causing B?'

A particular type of cause that often interests clinicians involves harm caused by the treatment they recommend. Simply put, questions of cause also include the question, does this intervention cause harm?

Research methods

There are essentially three ways of addressing questions about cause: descriptive studies (although these usually only suggest hypotheses about possible causes), case–control studies, and cohort studies.

Descriptive studies

This type of study describes things and includes some types of qualitative research. The descriptions often take the form of case reports or case series. Because there are no comparison groups in this type of research, it is difficult to draw clear conclusions about cause. However, these types of studies are very good at generating novel hypotheses that can be tested in other ways. An example is the report of eight patients with schizophrenia in south and southwest Finland in 1975 who developed agranulocytosis.[2] The authors suggested it might have been caused by the new antipsychotic, clozapine, that the patients had been taking – although agranulocytosis has many causes. Further research led to the finding that indeed this was the case, and that clozapine users needed special monitoring of their white blood cells. (A week after the first report the manufacturers of clozapine wrote to the Lancet suggesting that the high incidence of agranulocytosis in Finland 'points clearly to the possibility of a local factor' and that genetic, viral, and other possible causes were being investigated.[3] Two years later, in 1977, reports were still stating that 'there is no evidence that clozapine-related agranulocytosis is more common than the phenothiazine-related disorder'.[4])

Case–control studies

Case–control studies attempt to answer questions about cause by comparing a group of people with the disorder against a group of people without the disorder and examining in what ways they differ in exposure to a particular cause. A key aspect of case–control studies is that patients are enrolled in them on the basis of whether they have or do not have the disorder of interest. Figure 7.1 illustrates the basic design of a case–control study.

An example of a case–control study is that by Cheng et al.[5] that queried what factors play an important role in suicide. To do this, the authors gathered the records of 113 people who had committed suicide (the cases) and compared them with 226 people who had not committed suicide (the controls). The authors interviewed the families and asked about various risk factors including previous suicide attempts. They found that the incidence of previous suicide attempts (the exposure) was far higher in people who went on to commit suicide than in those who didn't. This is illustrated in Figure 7.2. The proportion of people who committed suicide who had a past history of suicide attempts was 24 out of 113 (21%) whereas only 9 out of 226 people (4%) who didn't commit suicide had such a history.

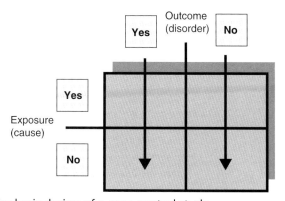

Fig. 7.1 The basic design of a case–control study.

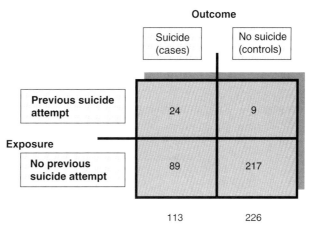

Outcome

	Suicide (cases)	No suicide (controls)
Previous suicide attempt	24	9
No previous suicide attempt	89	217
	113	226

Exposure

Fig. 7.2 A case–control study of risk factors for suicide.

Advantages and disadvantages of case–control studies

The advantages of case control studies are that they are quick and easy to do and they are good for rare outcomes. There are two main problems with case–control studies: firstly, in the choice of controls, and secondly, in assessing exposure. The cases are usually straightforward to collect as they have the outcome you are interested in. However, even here there can be difficulties in deciding who really is a case. For suicides it is sometimes quite hard to determine if people had intentionally killed themselves, and coroners may bring open or undetermined verdicts. A decision needs to be made whether to include such deaths or not. More problematic is the choice of controls. In the Cheng study, the authors chose to randomly pick their controls from the census records after they were matched for age, sex, ethnicity, and area of residency. The people who agreed to be interviewed may have been significantly different from those who did not agree, which may influence the findings. For example agreeing to be interviewed may have been associated with experience of the mental health system, so that the controls were more likely to have a higher incidence of psychiatric disorder and past suicide attempts, thus minimizing any difference with the cases. Alternative control groups that have been used in similar studies include those who make serious suicide attempts but survive and people who die suddenly through other means.

The second issue with case–control studies is the assessment of exposure. By definition, the outcome you are interested in has already happened when you do the study. This means that assessment of exposure to a risk factor is always retrospective. This can introduce bias if how you select your cases and controls also affects how assessment of exposure is determined. In the suicide study it seems reasonable to suspect that families of individuals who have killed themselves will be more likely to remember and give significance to events and behaviors indicating distress before the suicide than the families of people plucked at random from the census where no dramatic event has happened. This search to give meaning to a particularly distressing event is sometimes referred to as 'effort after meaning'. It can lead to significant recall bias where individuals with the disorder are more likely to remember or give meaning to events before an event than those who have not experienced the incident.

Odds ratios in case–control studies

The size of an association between an exposure and an outcome in a case–control study is described by the odds ratio. As its name suggests, this is a ratio of odds! Odds are defined as 'the probability, expressed as a ratio, that a certain event will take place'.[6] That is, the odds of an event is the number of those who experience the event divided by the number of those who do not. So the odds of flipping a coin and it coming up heads are 1:1 = 1, (even odds), because there are 2 sides of the coin and you are looking for only one of them; therefore, an odds ratio of one means that the event is equally likely in both groups.[7] The odds ratio can be a number from 0 (the event will never happen) to infinity. In the suicide example, the odds that someone who has committed suicide has a past history of previous suicide attempts is 24/89, that is 0.27 or about 1 in 4. The odds of someone who has not committed suicide having a past history of a suicide attempt is 9/217 or 0.04. The ratio of these two odds is 0.27/0.04, which is 6.75. What this means is that the odds of individuals who have attempted suicide eventually killing themselves are nearly seven times more than those who have not attempted suicide. Odds ratios are often hard to understand, although statisticians like them for their mathematical properties and casino operators for their ability to confuse. They are not the same as risk. In the example, the risk of someone who committed suicide having a past suicide attempt is 24/113 or 21% whereas the odds are 24/89, 0.27. One of the properties of odds ratios is that they always overestimate the real effect of an exposure to a cause.[8] This is more pronounced if the event rate in both the case and control groups is greater than 30% and the effect size is large (greater than a halving or doubling of risk). If the event rate is lower than this, and the effect size moderate, then the odds ratio will approximate to the relative risk.

To assess the importance of both odds ratios and relative risks, we need to know what the baseline risk is, as the odds ratio or relative risk tells you how the risk has changed relative to this risk. For case–control studies, the investigator determines the numbers of cases and controls, so the study design doesn't provide this information. Therefore, for case control studies the baseline or absolute risk often has to be found from other studies or from population data.

Cohort studies

Cohort studies attempt to answer questions about cause by following groups of people either exposed or not exposed to a potential cause. The number of individuals in each group who have the outcome of interest gives you a measure of the association between exposure and outcome. (The term comes from the unit of the ancient Roman army where soldiers served in cohorts – soldiers who died were not replaced and eventually the cohort was retired.) An important aspect of cohort studies is that subjects enter the study on the basis of their exposure to a potential cause (unlike case–control studies where individuals enter on the basis of having a disorder.) Figure 7.3 shows the design of a cohort study.

An example of a cohort study

A potential difficulty with prescribing lithium is the risk of causing birth abnormalities in the fetuses of pregnant woman taking the drug. To examine this question further, Jacobson et al.[9] enrolled 148 women who had been exposed to lithium during the first trimester of their pregnancy and compared them to 148 women who had not been exposed to lithium during pregnancy. (If this had been a case–control study, the design would have been to gather a group of women who had had babies *with* birth abnormalities and a group of women who had had babies *without* birth abnormalities, and then measure their exposure to lithium during their pregnancies.) They followed all these women through their pregnancies and recorded data on important outcomes such as prematurity and congenital defects in the baby. The results for all congenital defects are shown in Figure 7.4.

Here the proportion of women exposed to lithium who experienced a non-normal birth was 33/138, that is 24%, compared to 25/148, 17%, of women not exposed to lithium. This ratio 24%/17%, which in this case is 1.4, is known as the relative risk and means that women exposed to lithium in the first trimester are 1.4 times more likely to experience a non-normal live birth than women not exposed to lithium. (Note that the authors lost 10 women to follow-up so that their results are based on 138 women exposed to lithium not 148. This illustrates one of the significant problems of cohort studies, which is the difficulty of ensuring complete follow up.)

Advantages and disadvantages of cohort studies

The main advantage of a cohort study is that, because of the way it is designed, individuals are selected into the study before the outcome has happened. This means that there is less chance of the way individuals

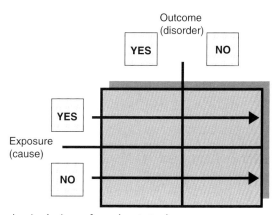

Fig. 7.3 The basic design of a cohort study.

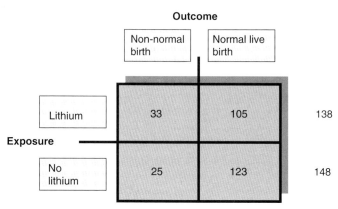

Fig. 7.4 A cohort study of lithium in pregnancy.

are selected biasing the outcome and that there is no problem with recall bias. This means that the results from cohort studies are usually more believable than from case–control studies. That is, they are a stronger design. Cohort studies are also good for rare exposures. The two main disadvantages of a cohort study are that it is more time-consuming and expensive to do than a case–control study, and there is a problem with being unable to follow people up over long periods of time, resulting in a higher risk of drop-outs and missing data (as demonstrated in the Jacobson study).

Relative risk

The strength of the association between an exposure and an outcome in a cohort study is expressed as the relative risk, which is simply the ratio of two risks. How this is derived has been explained in the example above, where the relative risk was 1.4. That is, the risk of pregnant women exposed to lithium having a non-normal birth was 1.4 times higher than nonexposed women. (Note that in this study the authors found that this difference could have arisen by chance (it was statistically not significant) so concluded that 'lithium is not a major human teratogen' and 'that women may continue lithium during pregnancy'. See Box 7.1 on the problem of interpreting studies which do not show a difference. The other advantage of cohort studies and the relative risk is that because of the design of cohort studies we can answer the question – 1.4 times higher than what? From this study we know that the risk in nonpregnant women is 17%, which makes the information clinically useful, and makes the risk in pregnant women about 24%, (1.4 × 17%).

Randomized controlled trials and assessing harm

Randomized controlled trials are usually used to ask questions about the effectiveness of different interventions. However, they can also be helpful in asking questions about harm. In this case, they can be

> **Box 7.1** The problem of interpreting studies that do not show a difference[10]
>
> Studies that do not show a difference between outcomes are relatively common in the literature. The lithium and pregnancy study by Jacobsen is an example of this. Here, the authors found that there was no statistically significant difference in the proportion of abnormal births between women exposed to lithium and those not exposed to the drug. The authors went on to conclude that prescribing lithium in pregnancy is safe. How believable is this statement? The issue is, were there enough women in the study for there to be a good chance of detecting a statistically significant difference? Consider the example of a bag of 200 marbles that contains 50 red marbles, 50 yellow and 100 blue. If you pick 'blind' 4 marbles out of this bag it is unlikely to represent accurately the ratio of the different colors in the bag. Even picking out 10 marbles is unlikely to represent the correct ratio of colors. To get an accurate impression you would have to pick out considerably more than 10 marbles. How many you need to pick out to stand a good chance of getting an accurate picture can be calculated beforehand by using what is called a power analysis. If this is not done until after you have picked out the marbles, you can calculate a confidence interval that will tell you how precise your estimate of the proportion of different marbles is. Clearly, the more marbles you pick out, the more likely you are to get an accurate measure of the proportion of marbles in the bag. The error of not detecting a difference when one really exists is called a type II error.
>
> So in reviewing the Jacobsen article we first looked for a power analysis – there was not one reported in the paper. Therefore, we looked at the confidence intervals around the main results. Here, we found that the relative risk for cardiac anomalies was 1.1 with a 95% confidence interval of 0.1 to 16.6. This means that in this study the risks of women who had taken lithium in pregnancy having babies with cardiac anomalies were 1.1 times greater than those women who had not taken lithium. However, the confidence intervals tell us that we can be 95% confident that the 'true value' of the relative risks is somewhere between 0.1 (in other words, lithium is protective) to nearly 17. Given this degree of uncertainty, and the potentially devastating effects of a bad outcome, we felt it was unwise to conclude, as the authors had, 'that lithium is not a major human teratogen'.

thought of as a special form of cohort study where the 'exposure' is randomly allocated to two or more groups of patients. This is informative where the harm is common. Where randomized controlled trials are not useful in assessing harms is where the outcome is rare but serious, for example suicide. In these situations the numbers in the trial are usually not large enough to detect any significant differences, and alternative research designs need to be used. Also see Box 7.2 on design terminology.

Critical appraisal of studies about cause/harm

Is the study likely to be valid?

1. **Were the patients and controls clearly defined?** The groups of patients need to be clearly defined so that we know to whom the causes apply and where there are likely to be biases. For example, in the suicide study we need to know if the suicides included just

---

Box 7.2 Prospective and retrospective: the confusing language of research

---

The words prospective and retrospective are often used to describe a research design. The reason they are used is that they indicate something about the quality of a study – prospective studies are supposed to be better than retrospective studies. This is because in prospective studies any exposure happens before the outcome, making them less susceptible to bias. This is true as far as it goes. Case–control studies are always retrospective. However, cohort studies may be either prospective or retrospective, depending on when the investigator does the research. Consider the question of low birth weight and its role in causing schizophrenia. One way to study this is to gather a group of babies, some of whom have a low birth weight and some of whom are of normal weight, and follow them for 40 years to see if they develop schizophrenia – clearly a cohort design. However, another way of doing essentially the same cohort study is to start with a population of people with schizophrenia in a certain geographical area. Then the investigator would get the birth records from 40 years previously of *everyone* born from the same area, divide them into low and normal birth weights, and see which of these babies went on to develop schizophrenia. The investigator is looking backwards in time, that is retrospectively, but the design is still a cohort study. For these reasons we try to avoid the terms retrospectively and prospectively, as they don't necessarily tell us important things about the quality of the study design. The terms 'cohort study' and 'case–control study' are far more informative.

---

coroner-defined suicides or open verdicts as well. Secondly, and importantly, were the cases and controls similar in all important ways apart from their exposure to the risk factor? The patients need to be similar in all respects apart from exposure to the cause to avoid biases and confounding. For example, in the lithium study it would be useful to know if the exposed and nonexposed groups had a similar obstetric history. If the exposed group also had a record of more stillbirths and spontaneous abortions, this would make them more likely to have subsequent problems.

2. **The question of measurement.** Were the exposures and outcomes measured the same ways in both groups? Was this measurement either blind or reasonably objective (for example death)? In the suicide example, the assessment of exposure was the same for both controls and cases and the outcome, suicide or not a suicide, was fairly clear. However, the investigators were not blind to the outcome. That is, they knew if they were interviewing the family of someone who had committed suicide or the family of someone picked at random from the census. This could bias the authors to finding more pathology in the suicide group, as this is what you would expect to find based on previous work.

3. **Was the follow-up of patients long enough and with few dropouts?** This is a problem with the lithium and pregnancy paper where we do not know what happened to ten of the women exposed to lithium. This makes analysis of the results difficult. One way of

dealing with this is to assume a worst-case scenario and put all the missing women in the 'worst' outcome. There is also an issue of length of follow-up in the lithium study. While it addressed the issue of congenital defects detectable at birth, it did not address the longer term consequences of exposure to lithium in pregnancy, as the babies were not followed up after birth.

4. **Do the results satisfy simple rules for causation?**
   - Is it clear that the exposure preceded the outcome?
   - Is there a dose–response relationship? In other words, is the outcome more likely to happen if the exposure is increased? For example, in the lithium study are women exposed to higher doses of lithium more likely to have non-normal births than women exposed to lower doses?
   - Is there evidence from a 'dechallenge–rechallenge' study? If the exposure is removed does the outcome stop, and if the exposure is then reintroduced does the outcome reappear?
   - Is the association consistent from study to study?
   - Does the association make biological sense? This is often the weakest test of causation, as our present state of knowledge of how the brain works is limited, which makes it relatively easy to make biological explanations that seem to make sense.

Are the results from this study important?

The size of the association between an exposure and an outcome is measured by either the odds ratio or the relative risk. The greater the number differs from 1, the greater the association. As has already been noted, importance depends on the baseline risk of getting the outcome. (For any odds ratio and baseline risk of outcome the number needed to harm (NNH) can be calculated from NNH=PEER (OR-1)+1/PEER (OR-1) (1-PEER) – where the PEER is the patients expected event rate, which can be estimated from the control event rate, and the OR is the odds ratio.)

Are these results relevant to an individual patient?

1. **Are the patients in the study so different from the patient that I am seeing that the results cannot be applied?** As mentioned previously, differences are in degree rather than absolutes. In other words, it is unusual for a particular patient not to be at risk from an exposure – what is more likely is that their risk may differ from those in the study.
2. **What is this patient's risk of the outcome?** The degree to which the patient's risk differs from those in the study is the subject of the next critical appraisal step. We can obtain estimates of risk from other studies, from the control group, or by using our clinical experience to estimate how our patient's risk varies. This is done in a similar way to working out how NNTs apply to individual patients as described in Chapter 4.

Last are two steps that apply if we are considering harms. Both follow the same process described in the section on relevance in Chapter 4 on treatment.

3. What is this patient's preference, concerns and expectations from this treatment?
4. What alternatives are available?

Searching for studies about cause or harm

For some questions about harm, randomized controlled trials of treatment are useful. This occurs if the harm is frequent and important, for example weight gain in studies of antipsychotics. If this is the case, then the Cochrane Database of Systematic Reviews or Clinical Evidence are likely to be useful. The advantage of these databases is that someone else has already done the hard work of synthesizing and critically appraising the relevant studies.

If the question is not about frequent and serious harms or is about causes, then a different search strategy will have to be used which doesn't involve randomized controlled trials. A quick way of accessing these for Medline is to use the Clinical Queries box in PubMed.

Clinical example 1

The scenario

One of us sees a patient who has a chronic paranoid schizophrenia that is reasonably well controlled by medication. The disorder takes the form of persecutory ideas that people around him are questioning his masculinity and are out to harm him. He had been told when he visited his GP that a new medication, quetiapine, might be better, as it was less likely to cause him to put on weight. He now wanted to try the new drug. The patient agreed, after much persuasion, to sit down and consider the evidence.

The question

In patients with paranoid schizophrenia, is taking quetiapine more likely to result in weight gain than olanzapine?

The search

This is a harm that is frequent and important and is likely to be reported in clinical trials of these drugs, so the first place we looked was the Cochrane Library. Entering the term olanzapine and quetiapine resulted in 17 systematic reviews that included these terms in the Cochrane Database of Systematic Reviews. Scrolling through these studies, there was none on delusional disorder but one on olanzapine in schizophrenia that had not been updated for two years and did not include any comparisons with quetiapine. There was also a systematic review on quetiapine in schizophrenia but this did not include any comparisons with other atypical antipsychotics. Looking in the Database of Abstracts of Reviews of Effectiveness (the DARE database) in the Cochrane Library using the same search terms, we found a 1999 article from the *American Journal of Psychiatry* on 'Antipsychotic induced weight gain'.[11] This review included 81 articles on the subject and found that in all the studies in which it had been measured, olanzapine produced a mean weight gain of 4.17 kg (95% confidence interval 3.7 kg to 4.64 kg) and quetiapine 2.49 kg (95% confidence interval 1.51 kg to 3.47 kg). As this is in the DARE database, it had already been critically appraised with the main comments that the quality of studies included was hard to assess and that how the studies were combined was not optimum. The authors of the critical appraisal wrote that the conclusions of this should be treated with caution. This is to some extent backed up by the authors of the article who wrote that weight gain is 'an incomplete, idiosyncratic and poorly defined matter'. At this point we could leave our search here and say to the patient that weight gain with these drugs is idiosyncratic but what little evidence we have suggests that weight gain with quetiapine is not likely to be greater than with olanzapine.

Alternatively, if time and resources permit, we could search harder. There are two ways of doing this. Firstly, we could search in Medline and Embase (Embase because this often includes drug studies not in Medline) for head-to-head comparisons of the two drugs in a randomized controlled trial where weight change is one of the outcomes. An alternative way of searching for the same information is to look in Science Citation Index and see where the *American Journal of Psychiatry* article is cited on the assumption that any studies since then on the topic will have cited this major review. First, searching in Embase entering olanzapine results in 3684 hits and quetiapine 1593 hits. Combining these there are 1227 articles that contain references to both these drugs. Unfortunately, in Embase there is not the option of limiting studies to those which are randomized controlled trials. What we did was to use randomized controlled trial as a search term (72 444 hits) and then combined that with the 1227 articles which referenced both drugs. This resulted in 47 hits. Scrolling through these articles, there are no relevant head-to-head trials of olanzapine and quetiapine, and in fact most of the articles are reviews that reference other randomized controlled trials. Next we searched Medline via PubMed. This showed 1559 hits for olanzapine and 505 for quetiapine. Combining these two terms and limiting the articles to those that were randomized controlled trials resulted in no articles being retrieved. Lastly, we entered the *American Journal of Psychiatry* review into Science Citation Index to find where this article had been cited. We found that it had been cited 207 times. We didn't have time to scroll through all these articles, but looking at the first 50 we found that most of the articles that had cited this paper were other reviews, mostly on drugs other than olanzapine and quetiapine.

So in this case, searching in the Cochrane Library we found the most relevant information with little effort with the advantage that it had already been critically appraised; searching in the other databases did not add anything to this. What we did in practice with this patient was to have a conversation about the advantages and disadvantages of changing medication. Whilst he wanted to try a medication that was less likely to put on weight he also wanted to avoid the anxiety of changing from a medication he knew worked to an untried one. The evidence we had was not compelling enough for him to choose a new medication. This led on to other discussions about managing weight and appearance, with the result that we were able to find some extra financial support for travel to the local pool to enable him to swim regularly.

Clinical example 2

The scenario

One of us has recently been involved in writing guidelines for the management of patients who present to a general hospital after deliberately harming themselves. Parts of these guidelines are recommendations on what sort of questions to ask. From our clinical experience it seems clear that a history of sexual abuse in childhood is common and relevant in such patients. However, we needed some evidence to back this up so we could recommend that clinicians always ask about sexual abuse as part of the initial history.

The question

In adults who deliberately harm themselves, is a history of childhood sexual abuse more common than in the general population?

The search

As this is a question about cause rather than about harms, databases that look only at questions about the effectiveness of therapies will not be relevant. This rules out Clinical Evidence and the Cochrane Library. Therefore, we began our search in Medline via PubMed, putting in the two concepts of deliberate self-harm and sexual abuse. Deliberate self-harm results in 3832 hits but, looking at how PubMed has done this search, this includes the text deliberate self-harm and the MeSH term self-injurious behavior but does not include attempted suicide. Searching on attempted suicide gets 7990 hits which when combined with the previous search term with OR (so that we get all articles that contain the concept deliberate self-harm or attempted suicide) results in 11 478 hits. Entering child abuse, sexual gets 4829 hits that combined with the self-harm search results in 142 hits. We only want to review papers that have a reasonable chance of being valid and relevant, so at this stage we searched these 142 papers using the term risk (which PubMed searches as the MeSH term and a text word), which narrowed down the articles to 54. (We also did the more extensive search recommended by Haynes et al. and this retrieved 68 of the 142 articles.) Scrolling down the first page of these 54 articles, we found an article by Coll et al.[12] on 'Abuse and deliberate self-poisoning in women: a matched case controlled study'. Fortunately, this paper was in the library, so we proceeded to critically appraise it.

Critical appraisal

Were the patients and controls clearly defined? The cases were women who had deliberately poisoned themselves, aged between 18 and 50, who were consecutive admissions to a hospital in England *and* who completed an abuse questionnaire. The controls were the next female admissions to the hospital for reasons other than deliberate self-harm.

Secondly, were the cases and controls similar in all important ways apart from their exposure to the risk factor? The first important difference between cases and controls was that all the controls approached completed the abuse questionnaire but only just over half (36 out of 70) of the potential cases completed it. This could introduce a bias that overestimates the risk of abuse. Women without a history of abuse could have been less likely to want to complete an intrusive questionnaire that is not relevant to them. Conversely, it could be argued that the study underestimates the amount of abuse in this population, as women with a history of abuse are less likely to be wanted to be reminded of it by taking part in this study. As 90% of the cases reported a history of sexual abuse, it is unlikely that the study seriously underestimates the incidence of abuse.

Next, the authors tried to match cases and controls for age, ethnic origin, social class, marital status, and area of residence. However, only 21 of the 36 cases could be matched with a suitable control during the period of the study. (This illustrates the problem of matching as a solution to confounding. Realistically most studies can only match on two or three variables before they run out of suitable controls.) This means that out of a potential 70 cases only 21 (30%) were included in the study – a potential for a serious bias in the selection of cases for this study.

The authors try to reassure readers that the differences between the matched, unmatched, and remaining cases are not significant by comparing the three groups on a number of different variables and finding no statistical difference between any of the information they collected. Most importantly, they record that the incidence of reported abuse in the 70 consecutive cases was 81%, which is not statistically significantly different from the 90% reported in the 21 women in the study (although how they found out about the history of abuse in the larger group is not recorded).

Next is the question of measurement. The history of abuse was measured the same way in both groups by way of a self-reported questionnaire. This method of recording exposure to a cause is subject to the problem of recall bias and is one of the major problems with most case–control studies. However, there is probably no way around it in this study. (Also, in this particular study it is possibly the memory of abuse that is important.) An interview by someone who did not know if the woman was a case or a control would have been better but more expensive, although it may have resulted in more women agreeing to do the study.

Was the follow-up of patients complete and long enough? The question of completeness of follow-up of patients does not really apply in this study. The average age of patients in the study was 34 years old, which clinically seems long enough for the consequences of childhood sexual abuse to have an impact.

Do the results of the study satisfy some tests for causation? Firstly, in this study it seems clear that exposure (childhood abuse) preceded the outcome (deliberate self-poisoning). Secondly, is there a dose–response gradient? In this study the odds ratios of someone who had been psychologically or physically abused going on to deliberately poison themselves as an adult was 1.02 and 1.05, respectively. The odds ratio of someone who had been sexually abused going on to harm themselves was 6, which makes the results more believable (assuming that sexual abuse is 'worse' than physical and psychological abuse). It also appeared that intrafamilial abuse was more likely to lead to later self-harm than extrafamilial abuse, again fitting in with what we would expect, given our knowledge of the effects of childhood abuse. There is no opportunity in this example for a dechallenge–rechallenge test of causation. The association between childhood sexual abuse and later self-harm seems to be consistent across different studies, although prior to this study all the other work had been on populations of women who had been abused (rather than women who had self-harmed). Does the association make biological or psychological sense? Our knowledge of how experiences as children affect us biologically as adults is still only at a rudimentary stage. However, problems in adulthood caused by abusive relationships as children would certainly be predicted by attachment theory.

Are the results important? The authors found that the odds of women self-poisoning who had experienced childhood sexual abuse is 15 times that of patients who had not reported sexual abuse (95% confidence interval 2 to 113). The very wide confidence interval tells you that the numbers in the study were small. In case–control studies, because of their problems with bias, we normally start to sit up and take notice when the odds ratio gets above 3, which is the case here. Note that there is a trade-off here between the size of the increased risk and the clinical importance of the outcome. Our threshold for the importance of the result depends in part on how clinically serious the outcome is. For example we are likely to pay more attention to a doubling of the risk of getting a myocardial infarction following exposure to a new drug than a quadrupling in the risk of getting a mild headache. One of the problems with odds ratios is turning them into something meaningful for clinicians and patients. There are two ways of doing this. First is to turn them into relative risks, which are much easier to understand. We can assume that the odds ratio is very similar to the relative risk if the rate of events in both groups is less than 30% and the effect size is moderate (a halving or doubling of risk). This, however, is not often the case with case–control studies where often at least half the individuals will have the disorder. (After all, one of the reasons for doing case–control studies is to get round the problem of rare outcomes.) The second way of doing it is to convert the odds ratios into numbers needed to harm (abbreviated to NNH). To do this, we need to know what the incidence of the outcome is in individuals not exposed to the cause we are investigating (also called the control event rate, CER, or the patient expected event rate, PEER). We can estimate this or find it out from the other studies. Looking at one of the references in this paper, we found it referred to a cross-sectional study of women drawn at random from the community in Otago in New Zealand, some of whom reported sexual abuse and some of whom did not. Examining this study, we found the rate of reported self-harm in nonabused adults was 0.4%. Using this figure we calculated that the number needed to harm was approximately 3 [1+ (0.04 × (15−1)/ (15−1) × 0.04 × (1− 0.04) = 2.9]. In other words, one extra person self-harmed as an adult for every third child who was abused compared to children who were not abused. (Reading through this example again, one of the issues it illustrates for us is the problem of turning feelings into numbers. By putting the incidence of child sexual abuse into a mathematical formula, it could appear that we are minimizing and ignoring the damage done by sexual abuse. We are not – sexual abuse is wrong and should not happen. However, this does not mean that we should not try to assess its impact.)

Exercises

1. The parents of a 26-year-old man with a six-year history of schizophrenia want to know if a head injury he had at 17 years old, when he fell off the back of a truck and was concussed, contributed to his disorder. Search in Medline for papers relevant to this question.

2. One of the papers you should find is by Nielsen et al. 'Is head injury a risk factor for schizophrenia'.[13] The authors describe this as a case–control study with 8288 people who have schizophrenia and 82 880 people without schizophrenia in the study. Who are the cases and who are the controls? In this study, what factors would you like to see controlled for?

3. The authors found that of the 5179 men with schizophrenia in their study, 280 had been concussed prior to their first admission for schizophrenia compared to 3201 men out of 51 790 without schizophrenia. Draw a two-by-two table to illustrate these findings. Calculate the odds ratio for concussion causing schizophrenia.

4. The authors of the paper found that this odds ratio was statistically significant. What does this mean? What does this odds ratio mean in words? What would you tell the parents of the man with schizophrenia about the role of concussion in causing his disorder?

Answers

1. We searched Medline using PubMed (free from anywhere). We used the following search strategy and found 18 papers relevant to the problem (see first table on p. 94). The search history is read from bottom to top – that is the way it is displayed in PubMed with the most recent search term at the top.

2. The cases are people with schizophrenia and the controls are people without schizophrenia. Note that this is a case–control study so that people get into the study depending on whether they have the

5	Search #3 **AND** #4	22:17:47	18
#4	Search **risk**	22:17:23	563 549
#3	Search **#1 AND #2**	22:17:11	239
#2	Search **head injury**	22:16:04	69 931
#1	Search **schizophrenia**	22:15:33	53 568

outcome you are interested in or not. (If this was a cohort study then people would be selected on the basis of whether they had been concussed or not.) Reasonable things to control for would be age and sex, as these factors are associated with both the onset of schizophrenia and the risk of having head injuries. In this particular question, it could be argued that given the often lengthy prodrome of schizophrenia, this may put individuals at risk of concussion by poor judgment leading to risky situations. Any difference that then arises between groups with or without schizophrenia may then just represent the effect of any prodrome. A clever way the authors got around this problem was also to record the number of nonhead fractures as a way of controlling for this phenomenon. (If the prodrome led to more accidents in general, then this would be reflected in a rise in other fractures, for example leg or arm, which would be unlikely to directly contribute to the cause of schizophrenia.)

3. A two-by-two table would look like this:

	Schizophrenia	No schizophrenia
Concussion	280	3201
No concussion	4899	48589
Total	5179	51790

The odds of someone with concussion having schizophrenia is 280/3201 (=0.087) and the odds of someone without concussion developing schizophrenia is 4899/48 589 (=0.1). Therefore, the odds ratio is 0.087/0.1, which is 0.87.

4. When the authors say that the odds ratio is statistically significant they mean that an odds ratio of this magnitude is unlikely to have arisen by chance. 'Unlikely' is conventionally taken to mean that there is less than a one in twenty chance of this ratio arising just by chance. Note that the larger the study, the more likely it is that the researchers will find statistically significant results.

In this context, what an odds ratio of 0.87 means in words is that the odds of someone with concussion developing schizophrenia are 0.87 times those of someone who does not get concussed. In other words, people who have been concussed are actually less likely to develop schizophrenia than those who have not been concussed. We would tell his parents that being concussed prior to his schizophrenia is unlikely to be an important cause of his disorder.

References

1. Olsen J. Some consequences of adopting a conditional deterministic causal model in epidemiology. Eur J Public Health 1993; 3:204–209.

2. Idanpaan-Heikkila J, Alhava E, Olkinuora M, et al. Clozapine and agranulocytosis (letter). Lancet 1975; 2:611.

3. Griffith RW, Saameli K. Clozapine and agranulocytosis (letter). Lancet 1975; 2:657.

4. Anderman B, Griffith RW. Clozapine-induced agranulocytosis: a situation report up to August 1976. Eur J Clin Pharmacol 1977; 11(3):199–201.

5. Cheng AT, Chen TH, Chen CC, et al. Psychosocial and psychiatric risk factors for suicide. Case control psychological autopsy study. Br J Psychiatry 2000; 177:360–365.

6. The Collins English Dictionary. London and Glasgow: HarperCollins Publishers; 1998.

7. Deeks J. Bandolier article, Swots Corner: What is an odds ratio? Centre for Statistics in Medicine, Oxford. Online. Available: http://www.jr2.ox.ac.uk/bandolier/band25/b25-6.html 14 Jan 2003.

8. Davies HTO, Crombie IK, Tavakoli M. When can odds ratios mislead? BMJ 1998; 316:989–991.

9. Jacobson SJ, Jones K. Prospective multicentre study of pregnancy outcome after lithium exposure during first trimester. Lancet 1992; 339:530–534.

10. Altman DG, Bland JM. Absence of evidence is not evidence of absence BMJ 1995; 311:485.

11. Allison DB, Mentore JL, Heo M, et al. Antipsychotic-induced weight gain: a comprehensive research synthesis. Am J Psychiatry 1999; 156:1686–1696.

12. Coll X, Law F, Tobias A, et al. Abuse and deliberate self-poisoning in women: a matched case–control study. Child Abuse Negl 2001; 25:1291–1302.

13. Nielsen AS, Mortensen PB, Callaghan EO, et al. Is head injury a risk factor for schizophrenia? Schizophren Res 2002; 55:93–98.

8

What is going to happen to me? Prognostic studies in mental health

Introduction

Prognosis is derived from the Greek for foreknowledge. It means a forecast of the probable outcome of a disorder. We are often also interested if there are any characteristics of a person that make them have a good or poor prognosis. These may be demographic factors such as age or sex or some characteristic of the disorder such as acuity of onset.

Research methods

Studies that address the question of prognosis are really special versions of cohort studies. As there is no question about etiology, there is no comparison group – just a cohort of individuals with a disorder who are followed up for a period of time and their progress assessed. Sometimes different cohorts, made up of individuals with different prognostic factors, are followed up simultaneously to assess the impact of these factors on outcome. An example of a prognostic study is that of Aguero-Torres et al[1] who asked the question, 'What is the mortality rate and survival time for older patients with dementia?'. The authors collected a group of 127 elderly patients who had been diagnosed with dementia in a community in Sweden and followed them for five years. They found that 70% of patients with dementia had died after 5 years, with a mean survival time of 3 years. Patients who were female and younger (between 77 and 84 years of age) had a worse prognosis. In order to help answer the question, 'How does this compare to people without dementia?', they also followed a comparison group of 790 nondemented people. In this group, 35% died after five years with a mean survival time of 4.2 years.

Critical appraisal questions for prognosis studies

Are the results of the study valid?

1. **Firstly, we need to know if the sample of patients was representative of the sort of patients that clinicians would see in practice and are clearly defined.** This is often a problem with studies done in specialized clinics and tertiary referral centers, where the obstacles that people have to overcome to be seen in such centers means that they are often quite different from the wider group of such patients. An example is chronic fatigue syndrome patients. Here, most of the studies have been done in specialized settings, yet most patients with chronic fatigue syndrome are not seen in such clinics. Taylor et al.[2] followed a random community sample of 51 patients with chronic fatigue in the United States. They found that in contrast to previous studies done in secondary or tertiary care, prognosis was related to initial severity of the chronic fatigue and postexertional malaise and not illness attribution, duration, or age. The issue of definition is a common one for all studies. It is hard to know if a study is relevant to you and your client if the patients in the study are not clearly described.

2. **Secondly, we need to know if the patients are at a similar point in their illness.** The subject of patients being at a similar point in their illness is a particular issue for prognostic studies. One way of thinking about such studies is that they are like a race where everyone has to begin at the starting line at the same time and with the same handicaps. If this is not the case then it is hard to know what the result of the race should be. For example, interpreting the prognosis of depression by following a group of patients, some of whom have had one episode of mild depression and some of whom have had repeated episodes of severe depression needing inpatient treatment, would be very hard. Such cohorts where patients are recruited at the same stage of their illness are known as *inception cohorts*. Staging of the illness may be by the length of illness, severity of illness or as, in the dementia study, at time of diagnosis.

3. **Next, was the follow-up of patients sufficiently long and complete?** There are two parts to this. First, the follow-up of patients has to be sufficiently long for it to have some clinical usefulness. Answering a parent's question about what is going to happen to their son with schizophrenia over the next ten years is not going to be answered by a study that only follows people for 12 months. Second, enough of the patients have to be included in follow-up to make the results meaningful. As with all cohort studies, patients being lost to follow-up are a major threat to their validity. Patients who are not followed up and included in the results may be very different from those who are included. Journals such as *Evidence-Based Mental Health* have a requirement that at least 80% of the patients need to be followed up for a study to be considered for inclusion.

4. **Lastly, were the outcome criteria assessed in a way that kept the investigators 'blind' to the starting characteristics of the patients?** The reason for this is to stop the investigators' biases affecting the

results of the study. Outcome criteria that do not allow for interpretation by investigators, such as death or hospital admission, are less susceptible to bias. The study is also more believable if the people doing the outcome assessment do not know what patients were like at the beginning of the study.

Is the study important?

1. **Firstly, if the outcome is very unlikely to happen it is probably not important.** Clinicians have to balance the rarity of an outcome against its severity to decide if it is important. Mortality would have to be very rare indeed not to be important.
2. **Secondly, we need to know something about the precision of the estimates of prognosis.** This is where confidence intervals are useful. Because we are unable to sample everybody with a particular disorder, we will always be examining a subsample of the whole population. This means that just by chance, if we repeated the study with a different population of people with the disorder (a different sample in other words), it is likely we would get a different result. It is likely that this result will be similar to but not the same as other studies on this disorder. The confidence interval gives a range of values that we could expect to get if we repeatedly did the same study on different populations. In the dementia study, the 95% confidence intervals around the mean survival time of 3 years from diagnosis were 2.7 to 3.4. This means that we can be 95% certain that the true value for the mean survival is between 2.7 and 3.4 years – a range sufficiently narrow to be clinically useful.

Relevance

1. **Is the patient you are concerned about so different from the ones in the study that you cannot use the results?** As before, the usual task here is to estimate how different the client is from those in the study rather than to decide that the study does not apply.
2. **Will it make an impact on what you choose to tell your patient or on your patient's choices?** Clearly, this partly depends on what treatments you have to offer. Clients with good prognoses would need a lot of persuasion to start any treatment, while the balance of risks and benefits would be different in someone with a poor prognosis.

Searching for prognostic studies

Searching in electronic databases for prognostic studies involves first selecting the clinical condition you are interested in and then using search terms that particularly look for study designs likely to yield believable conclusions. Haynes et al. found that using the MeSH terms 'prognosis' or 'survival analysis' found about half of all articles on prognosis and only retrieved 3% of irrelevant articles – a strategy with specificity. Similarly, a more sophisticated strategy found 97% of all articles on prognosis but also about a quarter of articles retrieved were not relevant to prognosis – a strategy with high sensitivity. As we have indicated in earlier chapters, in PubMed there is the facility of using a search filter, which is a way of applying the search strategies developed by Haynes without having to remember the specific strategies. You can also choose whether to emphasize sensitivity (maximizing the proportion of all relevant articles with the drawback of retrieving many irrelevant ones) or specificity (maximizing the proportion of irrelevant articles not detected at the risk of missing potentially relevant articles). To access these strategies, click on the Clinical Queries heading in the sidebar on PubMed.

Clinical example

The scenario

A 20-year-old is in hospital having inpatient medical treatment for complications of her anorexia nervosa. This is the first time she has had to come into hospital for treatment. Her BMI (body mass index) is about 14. She has had two years of various treatments as an outpatient for this disorder. She has held down several jobs, but none for longer than two months. She wants to go into higher education but her parents think she is being unrealistic because of her eating disorder. Her parents are concerned about how they are going to manage to care for their daughter in the future and are in some despair that they will always have her at home. They all want to know from you what is likely to happen in the future.

The question

In young women with anorexia nervosa, what is the prognosis and are there any factors which predict outcome?

The search

This search was done on PubMed at the beginning of 2003. First, searching for the disorder, anorexia nervosa, using the MeSH heading yielded 7327 hits. Next, as we were interested in prognosis, we entered the MeSH term Cohort studies, which includes the terms Longitudinal studies, Prospective studies, and Follow-up studies, as these are further down the MeSH hierarchy tree (Box 8.1). (PubMed automatically 'explodes' this hierarchy; in other search engines, cohort studies would have to be specifically exploded.)

This, when combined with anorexia nervosa, gave 554 hits. This is still too large a number to browse through, so we limited the search to English language publications (as these are likely to be more accessible to us) and to those articles with abstracts (this generally excludes letters and editorials). This gave 365 hits, still a large number. However, browsing through the first two pages we found a paper by Lowe et al. on the

---

Box 8.1   The MeSH hierarchy for cohort studies

Cohort studies

- Longitudinal studies
  - Follow-up studies
  - Prospective studies

long-term outcome of anorexia nervosa in a prospective 21-year follow-up study. This seemed to meet our needs and was available in our local library. (An alternative search strategy would have been to use PubMeds' Clinical Query function and use the built-in filters for searching. For a 'sensitive' prognostic search on anorexia nervosa, this yielded over a 1000 hits and a 'specific' prognostic search resulted in over 300 hits. We would then have had to reduce these numbers by restricting the hits to those that were English language and had abstracts.)

Critical appraisal   See Lowe B, Zipfel S, Buchholz C, et al. Long-term outcome of anorexia nervosa in a prospective 21-year old follow-up study. Psychological Medicine 2001 Jul;31:881–890.

Summary of results   Eighty-four women with anorexia nervosa were followed up 21 years after their first admission to a specialist eating disorders service. Seventy patients were still alive, of whom 63 (90%) completed the follow-up interview. The authors found that in this cohort 14 of 84 (17%) of patients with anorexia nervosa had died at 21 years follow-up (standardized mortality rate 9.8). Of the 14 dead and 63 living women, about half had fully recovered and 10% still met criteria for anorexia nervosa after 21 years. One in five were still living with family and three-quarters were able to work. A poor prognosis was associated with a low BMI on admission and greater psychological and social problems.

Is the study valid?   **Firstly, was the study representative of patients seen in clinical practice and were the patients well defined?** In this study the patients were recruited from a University Medical Hospital in Germany where they had been treated as inpatients for anorexia nervosa by a specialized eating disorders team between 1971 and 1980. Patients with serious medical co-morbidity were excluded. The 84 women in this study had an average BMI of 13.3 when first seen, with 43% showing bingeing and purging behavior and 57% showing restricting behavior and an average age of 21.

Patients were defined by the treating clinician using Feighner diagnostic criteria and retrospectively DSM IV criteria. Therefore, the patients in this study are reasonably well defined and representative of patients seen by specialist services (but not those seen in the community).

Was an inception cohort gathered? The patients were all at the stage in their illness when they were admitted to a specialist inpatient eating disorder service for the first time. This seems to us a reasonable and clinically useful way of ensuring that the patients in this study were at roughly the same point in their disorder.

Were the patients followed up for a sufficiently long time and were enough of them followed up? A strength of this study is that patients were followed up for 21 years and 90% of those still alive completed the follow-up interview.

Was the assessment of outcome blind or were objective measures used? The research team was blind to previous measures of outcome. Mortality, which clearly is an objective outcome measure, was also recorded.

Is the study important?   **Is the outcome likely to be common enough to be important?** The outcomes measured were full and partial recovery and various psychological and social outcomes that appear relevant to the clinical scenario. Mortality is a rare but important outcome.

How precise are the estimates of prognosis in this study? Unfortunately, the authors do not give any confidence intervals, although it is possible to calculate them from the information that they give. This is not practical for busy clinicians.

Is the study relevant?   **Is the patient in the clinical example so unlike the patients in the study that the results cannot be used?** The patient is being treated as an in-patient and has already had treatment in a specialist setting for two years. She is of a similar age to the patients in the study and lives in a similar developed country.

Will the results of this study alter the patient's or the parents' choices, or what you choose to tell the patient and her family? The results of this study can help the parents with a realistic appraisal of their daughter's future and help to adjust their expectations. It could also lead to a helpful discussion over the management of various prognostic factors.

Exercises

1. The strongest predictor of suicide is a previous episode of deliberate self-harm (attempted suicide). Describe how you would carry out a study to find out the prognosis of those people who had presented to hospital with an episode of deliberate self-harm. What difficulties do you anticipate?

2. Hawton et al.[3] describe a follow-up study of 11 583 patients who had presented to the general hospital in Oxford after deliberate self-harm between 1978 and 1997. They looked at mortality registers to find out if this group of patients had subsequently died and from what cause. Do you think that the authors gathered an inception cohort? Write down your reasons.

3. The authors found that 1187 people (about 10%) of the cohort had died by the end of 2000, of whom 300 (about 2.5%) had died by suicide. The risk was greater in men than women. However, the authors report that the risk of suicide one year after self-harm was 0.7% and after 5 years it was 1.7%. How do you explain the discrepancy between the overall study rate and the risks at 1 year and 5 years?

Answers

1. One way would be to gather an inception cohort of individuals who present to hospital after deliberate self-harm. The first difficulty would be in deciding who to include and exclude – only those who

take overdoses versus everyone; first-time presentations or everyone; native-language speakers only or not; and so on. The major difficulty would be in ensuring adequate follow-up so that people are not lost to the study.

2. This is an inception cohort, as everyone was at the same stage of their illness (they all started together). Important factors that may have 'handicapped' people, such as method of self-harm and previous history, were recorded to be factored into the analysis.

3. The discrepancy occurs because people were recruited into the study over 20 years (1978–1997) and the finishing point was the end of 2000. Therefore, people recruited in 1978 had 23 years to 'achieve' mortality whilst those recruited in 1997 only had 3 years. To take this into account when reporting prognostic studies, authors usually perform a survival analysis that takes into account the fact that some people have a much longer time to achieve an outcome than others.

References

1. Aguero-Torres H, Fratiglioni L, Guo Z, et al. Mortality from dementia in advanced age: a 5-year follow-up study of incident dementia cases. J Clin Epidemiol 1999 Aug; 52:737–743.

2. Taylor RR, Jason LA, Curie CJ. Prognosis of chronic fatigue in a community-based sample. Psychosom Med 2002 Mar–Apr; 64(2):319–327.

3. Hawton K, Zahl D, Weatherall R. Suicide following deliberate self-harm: long-term follow-up of patients who presented to a general hospital. Br J Psych 2003; 182:537–542.

9

Critical appraisal of psychiatric rating scales, diagnostic tests, and clinical decision rules

Rating scales in mental health appear attractive because they often seem to provide some certainty in a chaotic environment and remove some of the subjective aspects of assessment. They are used for a variety of reasons including screening for disorders, diagnosis, measuring change, and predicting future events. This chapter has several aims: firstly, to help users answer the questions 'is this a good rating scale' and 'what do the scores mean?'; secondly, to enable readers to critically appraise the literature on diagnostic testing, including using rating scales for case finding; lastly, to help clinicians ask powerful questions about rules that predict future events – especially relevant in mental health where there is so much emphasis on risk assessment.

Finding rating scales

Rating scales are marketed by several companies and are also available on the Internet. Some of the companies that market rating scales are M.D. Angus and Associates Ltd. (*http://www.psychtest.com/*), Psychological Assessments Australia (*http://www.psychassessments.com.au/*) and NFER Nelson (*http://www.nfer-nelson.co.uk/*). Users have to pay for these instruments and often have to register with these companies to prove that they will be using the scales in a professional capacity. The advantage of buying rating scales is that you can be sure that the copyright issues have been taken care of and that you get the proper instructions on use and scoring of the rating scales. The disadvantage is the cost involved. Increasingly, rating scales are also available on the Internet – some sites of which we are aware are described in Box 9.1. The instruments are usually free to download and reproduce but copyright and scoring is often unclear.

Box 9.1   Internet sites with access to rating scales

---

http://www.library.adelaide.edu.au/guide/med/menthealth/scales.html
University of Adelaide Library site with links to many sites with rating scales.

http://www.rcpsych.ac.uk/cru/honoscales/index.htm – site for the Health of the
Nation Scales (HONOS).

http://www.iop.kcl.ac.uk/IoP/Adminsup/Library/psy/topic2.shtml – Institute of
Psychiatry, Kings College, London.

http://www.alzheimers.org/chid/00000218.htm – several scales relevant to the
elderly.

To critically appraise rating scales, you need to be clear why you are
using them. The main reasons that people use rating scales are for diagnosis and predicting future events. Critical appraisal of rating scales
involves two steps. First is the appraisal of the scale itself, which broadly
addresses its conceptual background and feasibility of use. This step is
generic and common to all rating scales. The second step is the critical
appraisal of the studies that support the use of a particular rating scale,
and this is dependent on the use to which the scale is going to be put.
These studies inform the psychometric properties of the scale and focus
on validity and reliability.

Generic critical appraisal of screening rating scales

The first and most important part of appraising the usefulness of a rating scale is to ask, what is it for? The most common uses of rating scales
in mental health are for diagnosis, measuring change, assessing the
severity of a disorder once it is diagnosed, or for screening (Box 9.2). An
instrument which is designed for making a diagnosis is not necessarily
good at reflecting changes in the severity of a disorder. Consideration
also needs to be given to what settings the instrument was designed to
be used in; for example, whether in outpatients or inpatients and in
which cultural groups. The feasibility of using the scale also needs to be
considered; for example, some instruments require complicated scoring
schemes which may not be possible in clinical practice (see also Box
9.3). Other considerations are: training needed to complete the scale or
interpret the results; the scale acceptable to patients; the scale available;
and any issues with costs and copyright.

Second is the issue of the conceptual base of the rating scale. Rating
scales which assess the same disorder may have different conceptual
backgrounds. Snaith reviewed depression rating scales and described the
differences in the composition of the different scales and diagnostic systems.[1] The Hospital Anxiety and Depression Scale (HAD), for instance,
relies heavily on the concept of anhedonia with 85% of the questions
on this topic; the Beck Depression Inventory has only 14% of its items
on low mood and anhedonia, a third on hopelessness, low self-esteem
and guilt, and another 14% on appetite, weight and libido changes.

Box 9.2   Screening in mental health

Another common use of rating scales is as a screening tool; that is, a group of people who have either not presented to mental health services or have presented with some other problem are given a rating scale to see whether they are 'cases' of a particular disorder. This is not the same as screening in other branches of medicine where individuals *without* symptoms are 'screened' with some test which makes an early diagnosis, for example PAP smears in the early diagnosis of cervical cancer. In mental health, the process is akin to 'case finding' where people with symptoms are diagnosed when the correct test (often just asking the right questions) is performed.

The following guides help to answer the question whether screening or case finding does more good than harm.

- Does early diagnosis or case finding lead to improved quality of life?
- Are the people found through early diagnosis willing to take part in treatment?
- Is the effort taken in confirming the diagnosis made by the rating scales time and energy well spent?
- Does the frequency and severity of the disorder warrant the effort in early detection or case finding?

These scales reflect their authors' different views on depression and the uses of the scales. The Hospital Anxiety and Depression (HAD) scale was designed to detect depression in medical outpatients, while the Beck Depression Inventory was designed to assess the severity of depression in individuals already diagnosed with the disorder.

Box 9.3   Numbers in measurement

Rating scales by their very nature assign numbers to responses. There are several assumptions involved in doing this, not all of which are explicit. There are four ways in which numbers are used in measurement and we will briefly describe them.

Categorical – here numbers are assigned to categories, for example male=1 and female=2. It does not make sense to add, subtract, multiply, or divide these numbers.

Ordinal – numbers are assigned to responses that reflect some sort of hierarchical order. So on the HAD the response, 'definitely' to the statement 'I have lost interest in my appearance', is scored as 3, whereas the response 'I may not take care quite as much' is scored 1. We can say that 3 is clearly worse than 1. However, we cannot say that it is three times worse – in reality it may be twice or ten times worse. We cannot assume that the interval between each number on a scale is the same. Strictly speaking, we cannot add, subtract, or multiply numbers from rating scales. However, this is usually ignored.

Interval scales – here the interval between each number on a scale is the same but there is no true zero. An example is degree Celsius where 10 degrees is not twice as warm as 5 degrees (zero is just an arbitrary point on a scale). Numbers may be added and subtracted but not multiplied or divided.

Ratio scales – here there is a true zero. An example is height, where four centimeters is twice as high as two centimeters and the interval between numbers is the same.

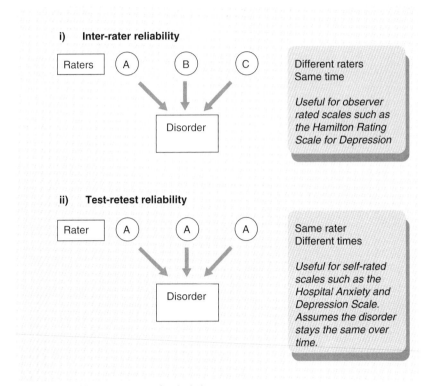

Fig. 9.1 Different types of reliability.

Reliability

The reliability of a scale is the degree to which scores can be replicated. Ideally, a good rating scale would give the same score for the same disorder at different times and with different raters. Conversely, a poor rating scale would give different scores if used by different raters at the same time to rate the same disorder. Two commonly reported types of reliability are illustrated in Figure 9.1. Both test-retest and inter-rater reliability are measured by a reliability coefficient, (either Pearson or an intra-class correlation), which should be above about 0.70.

A further measure of reliability is the internal consistency of the scale. For example, if a rating scale is designed to measure anxiety, it would be expected that people who score highly on questions about feeling panic should also score highly on questions about experiencing a racing heart. This is the internal consistency of the scale and is often affected by whether the instrument measures different concepts or the way the questions are worded. Measurement of the internal consistency is usually by a statistical measure called Cronbach's alpha, which has a range from 0 to 1, again values above 0.70 are considered acceptable[2].

Validity

The validity of a rating scale is its ability to measure what it is intended to measure. There are several types of validity, the main ones being face validity, criterion validity, and construct validity.

Face validity	The face validity of the scale is, quite simply, whether it looks as though it is asking the right questions. For instance, a scale asking about depression might ask about suicide but would be unlikely to ask about height. Note that good face validity is not always advantageous, especially when respondents may intentionally falsify answers to obtain some desired outcome.
Criterion validity	The criterion validity of a rating scale is the degree to which the test correlates with other accepted measures of the disorder, that is with other criteria. There are two types of criterion validity. Concurrent validity compares the correlation between the scale and other accepted measures at the same time. For example, a scale which attempts to diagnose depression should correlate highly with diagnoses derived from a clinical interview by experienced clinicians (a so-called 'gold standard') performed at the same time. Predictive criterion validity measures the correlation of a scale with some outcome in the future. Therefore, a scale which is said to predict suicide attempts, such as the Buglass Risk of Repetition Scale, should correlate with future episodes of deliberate self-harm.
Constructional validity	Constructional validity refers to tests which support hypotheses (or constructs) that can be derived from a rating scale. For example, with depression rating scales we can predict that people who score highly on these scales are more likely to be suicidal, receiving treatment, or to be disabled in some aspect of their daily lives. All these are hypotheses or constructs which we can test. A depression rating scale where high scores does not correlate with suicidality, for example, is unlikely to be a good measure of depression and therefore has poor construct validity. When we read studies that suggest that rating scales can be used as diagnostic instruments (Box 9.4) or to predict some future event, we need to critically appraise these studies (Fig. 9.2). The next section describes critical appraisal questions for these two uses of rating scales but they can also be applied to any other type of diagnostic test, such as CT scanning for Alzheimer's disease.

Critical appraisal of diagnostic tests

Are the results of the diagnostic study valid?	1. **Was the test compared with an independent, blind, reference ('gold') standard?** For rating scales, this is a test of criterion validity. The comparison should be with a test which is done independently of the new test, and the people doing the rating of the old and new tests should be blind to each other's results. The major issue in mental health is agreeing on what the reference standard should be. In other areas in medicine, tests can be compared with pathological changes in the body, whereas in mental health this is generally not the case (although there are some exceptions, Alzheimer's being an example). Generally, in mental health, for diagnostic tests the reference ('gold standard') is a clinical interview with an experienced clinician who is

---

Box 9.4   Diagnosis in mental health

Diagnosis is controversial in mental health. For some people, diagnosis means biological reductionism and the 'medical model'. This results in people being treated as objects who have lost their individuality and reinforces power imbalances. While there is some merit in these arguments we disagree that 'diagnosis' is unhelpful. Diagnosis is a form of classification and as such is inevitable and helps communication. The argument is that in any group of people, clients of a mental health system for example, we can recognize three types of characteristics. First, there are those characteristics which are unique to each individual, for example their life history or their genetic code. In this situation everyone is different and there is no point in classification as every individual is in their own special group. Second, there are those characteristics which everyone shares. Everyone has two parents, or lives in the same country for example. Again there is no point in classification as there would only be one group. Third are those characteristics which are shared by some but not all people. For example, some people may have blue eyes and some brown; some people may experience auditory hallucinations and some not. Once this third state is recognized, classification is inevitable – blue-eyed people and brown-eyed people – so the only argument becomes what sort of classification is most useful.

In psychiatry as in the rest of the medical field, there is a system of diagnosis which is useful for telling us and our clients something about how to manage their distress and what may happen to them in the future. What is different in psychiatry is that diagnosis is based on symptoms rather than cause, unlike the rest of medicine. In mental health we talk about depression not 'postloss disorder', whereas cardiologists make a diagnosis of myocardial infarction rather than 'central crushing chest pain disorder'. The reason for this is that the brain is far more complicated than the heart, is protected by a bony box and is indispensable for life. We simply do not know much about how the brain works and how it affects our behavior, feelings and thoughts. Classification by symptoms is less powerful than classification by cause, which makes diagnosis less important in mental health than in other settings. However, diagnosis is still inevitable, useful for communication, and does tell us and our clients something useful.

---

often guided by a standardized comprehensive interview (such as the Schedule for Clinical Assessment in Neuropsychiatry or SCAN). An example of a study to validate a rating scale is that by Zigmond and Snaith who designed the Hospital Anxiety and Depression scale to diagnose depression in medical outpatients.[3] Here, the authors asked 100 adults aged 16 to 65 who were attending medical outpatient clinics to complete the HAD. After each patient had completed the scale, they were interviewed by the researchers who made an assessment of the level of anxiety and depression without knowing the scores on the self-rating scales. The researchers were experienced clinicians but the criteria they used for making the diagnoses and assessing the severity of symptoms are not explicitly stated in the paper. This makes it hard to know what standard the scale was being compared with as well as making duplication of the study difficult. (However, since the original study there have been over 20 papers reporting on the use of the HAD that have used a variety of 'gold standards' including the Structured

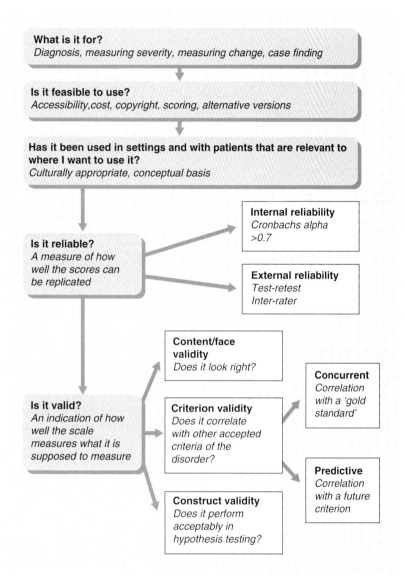

What is it for?
Diagnosis, measuring severity, measuring change, case finding

Is it feasible to use?
Accessibility,cost, copyright, scoring, alternative versions

Has it been used in settings and with patients that are relevant to where I want to use it?
Culturally appropriate, conceptual basis

Is it reliable?
A measure of how well the scores can be replicated

Internal reliability
Cronbachs alpha >0.7

External reliability
Test-retest Inter-rater

Is it valid?
An indication of how well the scale measures what it is supposed to measure

Content/face validity
Does it look right?

Criterion validity
Does it correlate with other accepted criteria of the disorder?

Concurrent
Correlation with a 'gold standard'

Predictive
Correlation with a future criterion

Construct validity
Does it perform acceptably in hypothesis testing?

Fig. 9.2 Is this a good rating scale?

Clinical Interview for DSM-IV diagnosis and several other rating scales.[4]) The authors found that there was a correlation between the interview scores and rating scale of 0.70 and 0.74 for the depression and anxiety subscales, respectively.

2. **Was the new test evaluated in an appropriate range of patients?** This is important as it is usually straightforward to distinguish between florid cases of a disorder and normal people (most people do not mistake a mouse for an elephant!). In these circumstances there is usually no need for a diagnostic test. A useful diagnostic test or rating scale needs to be trialed on people with a range of different severities of the

disorder as well as on people who have disorders which are often confused with the diagnosis you are interested in. So a test for Alzheimer's disease needs to be trialed on people with mild, moderate, and severe forms of the disorder as well as individuals with, for example, delirium (which is often confused with Alzheimer's). In the Zigmond and Snaith paper it seems that there was an appropriate range of severity of depression in the 100 people who completed the HADs with 12 people being diagnosed by the clinicians as having definite depression of varying severity and 22 people with borderline depression.

Are the results of the diagnostic test important?

To answer this question we need to understand sensitivity, specificity, predictive values, and likelihood ratios. To understand these ideas it is useful to draw a 2 × 2 table with the diagnosis or outcome along the top and the diagnostic test result along the side as in Figure 9.3.

If we put the results from the Zigmond and Snaith study into this table it can tell us several things (Fig. 9.4). Firstly, the proportion of people who have depression who score above the threshold of 11 or more on the HAD is 66% (8/12). This proportion, the number of patients with the disorder who score positively on a test, is known as the 'sensitivity' of a diagnostic test. Secondly, we can see that more impressively the proportion of people without depression who scored below the threshold on the HAD is 94% (83/88). This proportion, the number of people without the disorder who score negatively on a test, is called the 'specificity' of a diagnostic test. The sensitivity and specificity, while they are widely quoted, are of limited usefulness to clinicians. This is because as clinicians we see people who may or may not have a disorder – in other words, we work horizontally across the table rather than vertically. Sensitivity refers to a population of people all of whom have the disorder and specificity refers to a population where no-one has the disorder.

To address this issue, what we need to know is when a test result is positive what proportion of patients will really have the target disorder, and conversely when a test result is negative what proportion of patients really will not have the disorder. These two proportions are called, respectively, the positive and negative predictive values (often abbrevi-

		Disorder		
		Present	**Absent**	Totals
Diagnostic Test	**Positive**	a	b	a+b
	Negative	c	d	c+d
	Totals	a+c	b+d	a+b+c+d

Fig. 9.3   A 2 × 2 table for a diagnostic test.

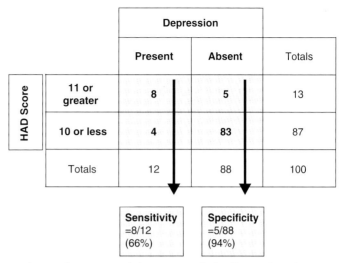

Fig. 9.4 The performance of the HAD scale in diagnosing depression – sensitivity and specificity.

ated to PPV and NPV). In Figure 9.5, the positive predictive value is 62% (8/13) and the negative predictive value is 95% (83/87). This means that if someone scores 11 or more on the HAD scale, approximately six times out of ten they really will have depression; similarly, if someone scores 10 or below then we can be pretty sure they do not have depression as only 5% (100% – 95%) or 1 in 20 people are misdiagnosed by a low score.

As one of the major uses of rating scales in psychiatry is for case finding, the positive and negative predictive values can give us important information. It is important to note that the positive and negative predictive values are affected by the prevalence of the disorder in the population. In Figure 9.4 the prevalence of depression in this population is 12% (12 out of 100 people surveyed had depression). However, if we increase the prevalence to 25%, which it may be following a myocardial

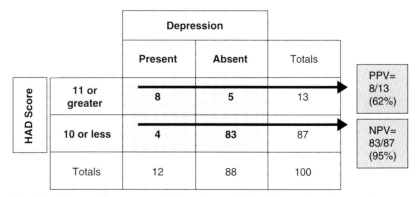

Fig. 9.5 The performance of the HAD scale in diagnosing depression – positive and negative predictive value.

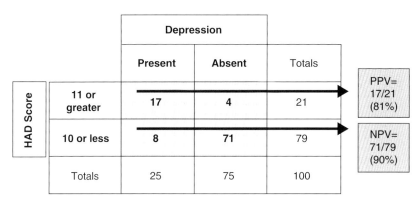

Fig. 9.6   The performance of the HAD scale in diagnosing depression – positive and negative predictive value. Prevalence of 25%.

infarction for example, the table changes as shown in Figure 9.6. Here, the sensitivity and specificity are unchanged. (They are proportions based on populations of individuals with and without the disorder, respectively, and we have not changed these except for changing their size. In Figure 9.6 they remain at about 66% and 94%.) The positive predictive value increases from 62% to 81% and the negative predictive value drops to 90% from 95%. When the prevalence increases, the positive predictive value increases, and as the prevalence decreases, the negative predictive value increases. For example, Meakin,[5] in reviewing the performance of self-rating scales in screening for depression in medical populations, found that for the Beck Depression Inventory the positive predictive value varied from 39% to 80% in populations where the prevalence of depression ranged from 12% (renal dialysis patients) to 59% (medical outpatients).

Likelihood ratios

Another interpretation of diagnostic tests involves the use of likelihood ratios. A likelihood ratio is the ratio of the probability of an abnormal test result in those with the disorder compared to the probability of the same test result in those without the disorder. In Figure 9.6 the probability of an individual with depression having an abnormal HAD score is 17 out of 25 or 68% (this is the sensitivity). The probability of someone without depression having an abnormal score is 4 out of 75 or 5%, (that is 100% minus specificity). Therefore, the likelihood ratio is 68% divided by 5%, which is 13.6. This means that an abnormal score on the HAD is 13.6 times more likely in someone with depression than in someone who is not depressed. Similarly, the likelihood ratio of a negative test result is 32% divided by 95% which is 0.33. In other words, a normal score on the HAD scale is about three times more common in those without depression compared to those with depression. Likelihood ratios are used to assess the importance of diagnostic tests (including rating scales), signs, and symptoms. If the likelihood ratio is high, say greater than 10, it can used to rule in the disorder. If the ratio is low, below 0.1, then it can rule out the disease. If the likelihood ratio is around 1, the test is likely to be uninformative and it is not worth doing. Therefore, if the HAD score is 11 or above, the individual is quite likely to be depressed and we need to confirm this by talking to the person. However, if the score is normal the situation is not so clear and we would have to do other investigations to decide if the person was depressed.

There are two problems with using likelihood ratios. The first is that to generate the post-test probability of someone having a disorder we need to know the pretest probability of the disorder. This information is rarely available and essentially relies on clinicians' estimates. Other ways of assessing pretest probabilities are: to develop practice databases that count the number of patients presenting with the same clinical problem, for example disturbed sleep, and report the frequency of disorders, such as depression, in those patients; to use the pretest probabilities in studies which assess the use of a diagnostic test; and to find studies specifically designed to assess the pretest probabilities of different diagnoses for a specific set of symptoms and signs. The second problem with likelihood ratios is that to make the post-test probabilities meaningful for clinicians and patients, the results have to be converted from odds to probabilities, which involves some calculation.

Are the results of this diagnostic test relevant to a specific patient?

1. **Is the diagnostic test available, affordable and feasible in your clinical practice? Has it been used in a similar setting?** Ideally the test should have been designed to be used in a similar service to the one your patient comes from. If you are working in a community team, the test should have been developed on patients in this type of environment rather than in primary care or an inpatient unit. This is because the probability of different disorders varies depending on where a practitioner works. A nurse working on a crisis team is more likely to see schizophrenia than a nurse working in primary care. To see how useful a test is in different settings we can alter the prevalence of the disorder to see how it affects the predictive values or, if we are using likelihood ratios, we can adjust the pretest probabilities to see whether they affect the post-test probabilities in a way that alters our diagnosis or management.

2. **Can we generate a sensible estimate of our patient's pretest probability (or can we make a reasonable estimate of the prevalence of the disorder)?** We have already described some of the difficulties with estimating the pretest probability. The pretest probability is a property of the patient and depends on certain risk factors, for example, age and sex as well as other clinical findings. The prevalence of a disorder, however, is a property of a population and is often easier to estimate from national or regional databases or from previous studies done in similar communities.

3. **Will the resulting post-test probabilities affect our management and be helpful for the patient?** The consequences of any test may be undesirable, for example, poor prognosis, and labeling; it may lead to further tests using new pretest probabilities; or it may be good

news involving the absence of a disorder or a better prognosis. All these factors need to be considered along with the patient's values and needs when presenting for help. A systematic review of the use of rating scales for case-finding in nonpsychiatric settings[6] found that feedback of the results to clinicians made little difference to the recognition of psychiatric disorders. The exception was when only the results of high scorers was fed back to the clinicians; here, the rate of recognition increased but this still did not result in any increase in effective intervention or better outcomes for patients. The authors make the point that increased recognition and effective intervention is more likely to happen when 'feedback of individualized positive test results is accompanied by increased resources and local educational interventions delivered by opinion leaders'. The point here is that the context of the results of testing and the uses to which they are put are important in deciding their relevance and usefulness.

A project to improve the accuracy and completeness of reporting diagnostic studies is the STARD initiative. STARD stands for the Standards for Reporting of Diagnostic Accuracy and is the work of an international group who have produced a checklist of 25 items for studies that report diagnostic accuracy and a flowchart of a model study to assess diagnostic accuracy.[7]

Clinical decision rules

Sitting somewhere between prognosis and diagnosis is a particular category of tests that predict the probability of future events. These are particularly relevant in mental health, given the increasing clinical focus on risk and preventing suicide and homicide. Clinical decision rules are tools which gather information from diverse sources such as the patient's history, mental state, physical investigations, and from carers. This information is combined into a mathematical model that is used to predict important outcomes. Finally, the best predictors from the model are converted into a clinically useful algorithm which can be used without complex calculations. Examples from mental health are the Buglass Risk of Repetition Scale for predicting future self-harm,[8] tools that try to predict suicide, and rules for deciding which patients with early dementia should undergo neuroimaging to detect a reversible cause of dementia. The critical appraisal of clinical decision rules is similar to that of prognosis. Some authors have divided the critical appraisal of clinical decision rules into the appraisal of studies which derived the tool and studies which have validated the tool.[8] We have not done this, as we think the approach we describe is simpler and similar to other critical appraisal guides. Also, in practice often the same paper will present both the derivation and the validation of the clinical decision rules.

Are the results of the study valid?

1. **Was a representative group of patients, chosen in an unbiased fashion, followed up without significant drop-outs?** This is similar to the first guide in critically appraising prognostic studies.

2. **Were all potential predictors included in the derivation of the rule?** Deciding what to include in a model can be based on expert opinion or from previous studies that have investigated prognosis. Some authors include all feasible factors and rely on statistical techniques to test which are important. To make a clinically relevant tool, the predictors chosen should be present in a significant proportion of the population.

3. **Were the potential predictors considered individually as well as together?** What is important here is whether an attempt was made to see how the different predictors or risk factors interacted together. As clinicians, we know that different patients with the same diagnosis can have very different prognoses. Two patients with anorexia nervosa may have the same diagnosis but different prognoses depending, for example, on their initial BMI, history of bingeing, and history of treatment response. It may be that a low BMI and a history of poor treatment response doubles the risk of a poor outcome and that adding a history of bingeing to this does not increase the predictive power of the model. There are several mathematical techniques which can tell us how much individual risk factors predict the final outcome and how they interact with other risk factors. Fortunately, we do not have to understand the statistics behind them; our main task is to make sure that some attempt has been made to use them when deriving the model. The two most common techniques are some form of regression or discriminate analysis, and recursive partitioning.

4. **Were the potential predictors and the outcome variables clearly defined?**

Are the results of the study important?

1. **How well does the tool discriminate between those with good outcomes and those with bad outcomes? How precise are the estimates of risk?**

Is the tool relevant to your clinical practice?

1. **Is the tool feasible to use?** What is important here is that you have the facilities to use the tool. It is no good having a clinical decision tool that requires information from a CT scan if you do not have ready access to a scanner. Similarly, tools which rely on complex computer algorithms are unlikely to be used in clinical practice.

2. **Has the tool been validated in a new sample of patients?** We are likely to be more convinced of the relevance of a clinical decision rule if it can be demonstrated to be effective in different locations and in different groups of patients.

3. **Are your patients similar to those patients used in deriving and validating the tool?**

4. **Does the tool improve on your clinical decisions?**

An example of an attempt to derive clinical decision rules is a paper by Goldstein et al[9] where an attempt was made to produce a set of rules (or model) that would predict suicide. Firstly, they identified 1906 people who had been admitted to a psychiatric hospital in Iowa, USA, with a mood disorder. These people were chosen, as they would be expected to be at high risk of suicide. Next they identified 21 different variables which they thought may be predictive of suicide, including demographic features such as age and sex, historical information such as number of previous hospitalizations and number of suicide attempts, diagnosis, and current mental state. The authors identified the presence of the potential risk factors for each patient and then the patients were followed up for 13 years. At the end of the follow-up period, 46 patients who had died by suicide were identified by searching through the record of death certificates for the state. Then, using a statistical technique called multiple logistic regression they identified which of the 21 previously identified risk factors were statistically significantly associated with eventual suicide. These were sex, suicidal ideation on admission, bipolar disorder, outcome at discharge (favorable or unfavorable), unipolar depression with a family history of mania, and number of previous suicide attempts. However, when these risk factors were combined together to predict the suicides in the initial cohort the model failed to predict any of the 46 suicides that had occurred in the 1906 original patients.

So, using the critical appraisal rules, can we believe these results, are they important, and are they relevant? Firstly, was a representative group of patients chosen in an unbiased fashion and followed up without significant drop-outs? The patients chosen were all admissions to a psychiatric hospital in Iowa who also resided in the state. So there is unlikely to be any problems with representativeness or bias. They were followed up for up to 13 years but only the death certificates from the state of Iowa were examined. This means that it is possible that some patients had left the state and then committed suicide elsewhere and so would not be included in the final number of suicides. It is unlikely, however, that this would be a large number of deaths. Secondly, were all potential predictors included in the derivation of the rule? The answer here is yes, most of the risk factors included in the rule are those identified by other authors as important in predicting suicide. Thirdly, were the potential predictors considered individually as well as together? The authors used a multiple logistic regression analysis to see how the risk factors interacted, which is one of the usual ways of considering how the potential predictors interact. Lastly, were the potential predictors and the outcome variables clearly defined? The potential predictors were clearly defined using standard diagnostic criteria or common sense clinical measures. The outcome of suicide is always problematic, however, as there is often considerable uncertainty about what is counted as a suicide and what is not. Drownings and single-person car deaths, for example, are always hard for coroners to decide whether they are suicides or not. In this study the authors relied on death certificates rather than on personal follow-up of the patients, which would have led to an underestimation of the true number of suicides.

Next we need to consider if the results of the study are important. Here the questions are, how well does the tool discriminate between those with good outcomes and those with bad outcomes, and how precise are the estimates of risk? Unfortunately, in this study the model derived from the potential risk factors failed to predict any of the suicides. Paradoxically, this is probably an important outcome, as it indicates that in this area at least trying to predict those who will kill themselves is not worth doing, and efforts should be put into prevention (this is a subtle but very important distinction which is the basis of road safety campaigns and the efforts of the commercial airline industry to make flying safer than driving to the airport).

Lastly, are the results of this study relevant to our practice? Is the tool feasible to use? The risk factors in the tool are easily ascertained clinical variables which require no special techniques and should be part of any standard clinical assessment. Has the tool been validated in a new sample of patients? The authors validated the tool on the original group of patients. Given that it failed to predict any of the subsequent suicides, it would be hard to get funding to test this on a new group of patients or in different settings where patients are likely to be of lower risk.

Are your patients similar to those patients used in deriving and validating the tool? This tool was designed to be used for psychiatric inpatients and is most relevant to this group. Does the tool improve on your clinical decisions? In this instance, no!

Exercises

For the exercises for this chapter we will describe a study and then ask questions based on the paper, Brewin CR, Rose S, Andrews B, et al. Brief screening instrument for post-traumatic stress disorder. British Journal of Psychiatry 2002; 181:158–162.

Design

Validation study of a new brief questionnaire (The Trauma Screening Questionnaire [TSQ]) compared to a clinical interview (Clinician-Administered PTSD [Post-Traumatic Stress Disorder] Scale (CAPS-I).

Setting

Telephone interviews from a London specialist center.

Patients

Forty-one passengers (mean age 38 years, 51% men) from one of two trains that crashed at Ladbroke Grove in 1999. Patients having routine clinical follow-up after the crash were contacted by letter. Those agreeing to take part were included in the study: 18 out of 44 patients treated at St Mary's Hospital, London, and contacted: 15 out of 25 patients treated at the Royal Berkshire Hospital, Reading, and contacted; and 8 members (response data not available) of a survivors' group set up after the crash.

Intervention

TSQ administered by telephone. CAPS administered by telephone 1 week later.

Main outcome measure

Sensitivity and specificity for diagnosis of PTSD using different numbers of items from the TSQ compared to diagnoses made by CAPS.

Main results   Fourteen out of 41 (34%) responders received a CAPS diagnosis of PTSD. At least six re-experiencing or of arousal symptoms, in any combination on the TSQ, showed a sensitivity of 0.86 and specificity of 0.93. The findings were replicated on data from a previous study of 157 crime victims.

Conclusion   The TSQ is a brief, easy to administer scale that shows high sensitivity and specificity for diagnosing PTSD.

Questions
1. How useful is the scale?
    (a) What is it for?
    (b) What settings was the instrument designed to be used in?
    (c) Is training needed to complete the scale or interpret the results?
    (d) Is the scale acceptable to patients?
    (e) Is the scale available and are there any issues with costs and copyright?
2. Does case finding do more good than harm?
    (a) Does case finding lead to improved quality of life?
    (b) Are the people found through early diagnosis willing to take part in treatment?
    (c) Is the effort taken in confirming the diagnosis made by the rating scales time and energy well spent?
    (d) Does the frequency and severity of the disorder warrant the effort in early detection or case finding?
3. Are the results of the study valid?
    (a) Was a representative group of patients, chosen in an unbiased fashion, and followed up without significant drop-outs?
    (b) Were all potential predictors included in the derivation of the rule?
    (c) Were the potential predictors considered individually as well as together?
4. Are the results of the study important?
    (a) How well does the tool discriminate between those with good outcomes and those with bad outcomes?
    (b) How precise are the estimates of risk?
5. Is the tool relevant to your clinical practice?
    (a) Is the tool feasible to use?
    (b) Has the tool been validated in a new sample of patients?
    (c) Are your patients similar to those patients used in deriving and validating the tool?
    (d) Does the tool improve on your clinical decisions?

Answers

1. How useful is the scale?
    (a) To usefully screen people for those with a diagnosis of PTSD.
    (b) People who have been involved in a trauma.

(c) No training is needed to complete the scale or interpret the results.

(d) How acceptable patients found the scale is not presented.

(e) The scale is published with the paper and there appear to be no special issues with costs and copyright.

2. Does case finding do more good than harm?

(a) Treatments are available for people with PTSD but it is unclear whether case finding leads to improved quality of life.

(b) The study does not establish whether people diagnosed with PTSD will be willing to take part in treatment.

(c) The rating scale is quick to administer and requires no training.

(d) PTSD is common after major traumas.

3. Are the results of the study valid?

(a) The group of patients is not necessarily representative because only 48% of those contacted agreed to take part in the study. It is not clear if you can generalize from one trauma to another.

(b) No, only a small number of potential predictors were included in the derivation.

(c) Different numbers of items were used in the calculations.

4. Are the results of the study important?

(a) People with a diagnosis of PTSD are likely to have a poorer prognosis but this study does not demonstrate that.

(b) The 95% confidence intervals are not included, but the sample size is small so the estimates are likely to be poorly precise.

5. Is the tool relevant to your clinical practice?

(a) The tool is feasible to use because it is brief, does not require training and can be administered over the phone.

(b) The scale has also been validated on 157 crime victims. The findings need to be replicated on larger samples.

(c) Your patients are likely to differ from these patients unless they suffer a similar trauma in a similar setting.

(d) The tool does not necessarily improve on your clinical decisions.

References

1. Snaith, P. What do depression rating scales measure? Br J Psych 1993; 163:293–298.
2. Streiner DL. A checklist for evaluating the usefulness of rating scales. Can J Psych 1993; 38:140–148.
3. Zigmond AS, Snaith RP. The Hospital Anxiety and Depression Scale. Acta Psychiatr Scand 1983; 67:361–370.
4. Herrmann C. International experiences with the hospital anxiety and depression scale – a review of validation data and clinical results. J Psychosom Res 1997; 42:17–41.
5. Meakin BJ. Performance of self-rating scales in screening for depressive syndromes in the medically ill. Pschology 1992; 160:212–216.
6. Gilbody SM, House AO, Sheldon TA. Routinely administered questionnaires for depression and anxiety: systematic review. BMJ 2001; 322:406–409.
7. Bossuyet PM, Reitsma JB, Bruns DE, et al. Towards complete and accurate reporting of studies of diagnostic accuracy: the STARD initiative. BMJ 2003; 326:41–44.
8. McGinn TG, Guyatt GH, Wyer PC, et al. Users' guides to the medical literature XXII: How to use articles about clinical decision rules. JAMA 2000; 284:79–84.
9. Goldstein RB, Black DW, Nasrallah A, et al. The prediction of suicide. Sensitivity, specificity, and predictive value of a multivariate model applied to suicide among 1906 patients with affective disorders. Arch Gen Psych 1991; 48:418–422.

10

Critical appraisal of qualitative research

A common criticism of evidence-based medicine is that it is somehow against qualitative research. Qualitative research involves the process of describing in rich detail, but in a transparent way, various social and psychological phenomena. 'The goal of qualitative research is the development of concepts which help us to understand social phenomena in natural (rather than experimental) settings, giving due emphasis to the meanings, experiences, and views of all the participants.'[1] It is particularly suited to answering questions about how things happen. The paper referred to in Chapter one by Ely[2] on the obstacles to implementing evidence-based medicine is an example of qualitative research. Here, the task was not to test a hypothesis but, by careful observation and analysis of the behavior of family doctors, to describe a taxonomy of barriers to practicing evidence-based medicine. The qualitative and quantitative dichotomy has been exaggerated in the past and is unhelpful to the subjects it is supposed to help. A more useful way of thinking about these different approaches is that they complement each other. Qualitative research is good at generating hypothesis which may be tested with quantitative research; quantitative and qualitative methods can be used together to provide different types of evidence to support a hypothesis (research on life events is a good example of this); and finally, qualitative research can examine some things which are not amenable to quantitative methods, for example the experience of implementing change in complex health systems. It is unusual for a clinical question to be generated and answered in a single study. More usually, there is an evolving research process which may take decades of debate and study before any clear conclusions may be reached. Qualitative and quantitative research both have their place in this process. For example, a qualitative study on the experience of survivors of disasters may generate hypotheses around the importance of social networks in helping people. This may be incorporated into a treatment for trauma survivors, the effectiveness of which is tested in a randomized controlled trial. How the treatment is delivered in clinical practice and identifying barriers to its use may form part of a further qualitative study, and so the process continues.

Qualitative research is attractive to clinicians because it is often more feasible to do than quantitative research, and the skills of in-depth interviewing and identifying themes are familiar from clinical practice. There is also a considerable tradition of qualitative research in health care, and mental health is no exception. The classic phenomenologists of the 19th and 20th centuries described a series of qualitative studies on abnormal mental phenomena in great detail; Freud outlined his theory of the mind based on in-depth qualitative studies of a few patients. The boundary between case studies and formal qualitative research is at times unclear, although they are both used to answer similar types of the question 'what is going on and how could we explain it?' More formal qualitative research is transparent about how the subjects in a study are collected, and in some instances purposely selects a particular group of subjects to explore a certain territory. The method of data collection and the generation of hypotheses has also become more explicit and transparent. Data collection may be by interview, observation, written record, focus groups, or by a mixture where the process of triangulation describes the process of checking one method of data collection against another. The transparency often involves explicit recognition of the researchers' bias, power imbalances in the interview, and other differences. The analysis of data is an evolving methodology but essentially it involves generating a theory from the observed data. Particular techniques include grounded theory, interpretative phenomenological analysis, and analytical induction.[3] What most of these techniques have in common is that the researchers immerses themselves in the data, derives a hypothesis, and then tests the hypothesis on further cases until no new hypotheses emerge.

Another issue with qualitative research is finding it in electronic databases. It seems that CINHAL has more useful indexing terms for qualitative research[4] than Medline, but this has to be weighed against the much greater size of Medline. For now, it seems the best way to go is to search on words which indicate qualitative research such as 'grounded theory' as textwords in the major databases.

The issue of deciding whether a piece of qualitative research is 'good' or not is controversial. For those who are interested, Mays and Pope outline the arguments.[5] We feel it is important for clinicians to have some way of judging the quality of claims made in qualitative research, as with other types of research, so we have described some critical appraisal questions below.[6,7]

Is the research valid and transparent?

Here, it is important for readers of the research to be able to judge for themselves the validity of the arguments made by the authors. To do this, it is important that the authors present the methods that they used in a clear way. This should probably involve a description of how subjects were chosen for the study (the sampling strategy), how the data was collected, and whether it was done in a systematic way. An example of a qualitative study is that by Freeman and Sweeney[8] on the reasons why general practitioners do not always implement best evidence. The authors asked participants to participate in three focus groups where they were asked to discuss a case in which they had knowingly not followed evidence-based practice. The focus groups were recorded and transcribed by the researchers. Using a grounded theory approach, the authors identified six main themes which affected the implementation of evidence-based treatment. These included logistical problems, perceived tensions between primary and secondary care, and personal and clinical experience. The general practitioners were also aware that how they framed choices affected whether evidence was implemented. In this study, the systematic collection of the data is clearly described. The general practitioners are described as volunteers, but how they volunteered is not recorded. Next, any exceptions to the theory that the researchers have developed should be discussed. Ideally, the researcher should give some evidence of seeking out observations that might have modified the theory. Presenting data in qualitative research is problematic, as this can run to hundreds of pages of transcript. However, reports of qualitative research should include sufficient original evidence, such as quotes, to make a case for the link between the evidence and the interpretation. Finally, there should be some discussion of the effect of the researchers' presence on the research process and how that may have affected the data collected.

Is the study important and relevant?

Here the authors should state what the research question is and justify why they are asking it. In the Freeman paper, the authors clearly state that the aim of the study was to explore why general practitioners do not implement evidence-based treatments. The importance was justified by reference to the increasing interest in evidence-based medicine and the acknowledgement that implementing evidence-based approaches faces significant barriers. Next, the clinical implications of the study should be spelled out. In our example, the authors emphasize that doctors' personal and professional experiences and their choice of words affects whether evidence-based treatments are carried out. Lastly, there should be some statement about the reasons for choosing to use qualitative research for the particular research question. See Box 10.1 for a summary of critical appraisal of qualitative research.

Box 10.1 Critical appraisal of qualitative research

Is the research valid and transparent?

Were the methods described clearly?

How were the subjects chosen?

Did the researchers provide any evidence of seeking out observations that may have modified the theory?

Did the evidence presented make a case for the link between the evidence and its interpretation?

Was there any discussion of the researchers' presence on the research process and how that may have affected the data?

Is the study important and relevant?

Is the research question clear?

What are the clinical implications of the research?

Why use qualitative research to address this question? What advantages does qualitative research bring to the question?

References

1. Pope C, Mays N. Qualitative research: reaching the parts other methods cannot reach: an introduction to qualitative methods in health and health services research. BMJ 1995; 311:42–45.
2. Ely JW, Osheroff JA, Ebell MH, et al. Obstacles to answering doctors' questions about patient care with evidence: qualitative study. BMJ 2002; 324:710–717.
3. Fossey E, Harvey C, McDermott, et al. Understanding and evaluating qualitative research. Aust NZ J Psych 2002; 36:717–732.
4. Evans D. Database searches for qualitative research. J Med Libr Assoc 2002; 90:290–293.
5. Mays N, Pope C. Assessing quality in qualitative research. BMJ 2000; 320:50–52.
6. Brown C, Lloyd K. Qualitative methods in psychiatric research. Advances in Psychiatric Treatment 2001; 7:350–356.
7. Mays N, Pope C. Qualitative research: rigour and qualitative research. BMJ 1995; 311:109–112.
8. Freeman AC, Sweeney K. Why general practitioners do not implement evidence: qualitative study. BMJ 2001; 323:1100–1102.

11

What to do if there is no evidence

One of the major complaints about the process of solving clinical problems using the methods we have described is that often there is no evidence for the problem that you can believe or is relevant. This is particularly important with questions about the best therapy. The large randomized controlled trial of a particular treatment for a particular disorder may not have been done, the patients in the trials are not like your patients, or the disorder is so rare it is unlikely that a randomized controlled trial will ever be done. The question then arises, how do you solve these problems? Traditionally, the answer to this is that clinicians rely on their experience, knowledge of basic mechanisms (whether psychological or physiological), and clinical instinct. Clearly these all have their place. However, there are several well-described heuristics or 'rules of thumb' that clinicians use subconsciously that can seriously distort their decision making. Such biases in diagnosis include being more likely to make a diagnosis when instances of the disorder are easier to recall (the availability heuristic), and selectively gathering and interpreting evidence that confirms a diagnosis while ignoring evidence that might refute it (the confirmation heuristic). When deciding on different courses of treatment, clinicians tend to choose riskier treatments when they are described in negative (for example mortality), rather than positive (for example survival), terms (the framing heuristic) and will choose a given treatment option more often when there are additional alternatives rather than just one choice. Often clinicians will decide on a 'trial of treatment' where the patient is given a therapy and various clinical outcomes are assessed over a period of time. At some point the decision is then made whether to continue or stop the treatment. The difficulties with this common scenario are that it ignores the placebo effect and the natural history of the disorder; the expectations of the therapy by the patient and the clinician may influence the effectiveness of the treatment; and both clinician and patient may be motivated not to let each other down.

This chapter describes two methods of answering questions about therapy where there is no or limited evidence. The first are N of 1 trials, which are randomized controls in individual patients. The second is the process of decision analysis where constructing a model of a clinical decision and adjusting some of its parameters (a sensitivity analysis) can inform decision making in situations of uncertainty.

N of 1 trials

An N of 1 trial is a randomized controlled trial in an individual patient. It brings the benefits of randomization, especially controlling for bias and the placebo effect, to an individual's clinical problem. Although based originally on work in behavioral psychology, the main clinical application involves questions around drug treatments. The process of an N of 1 trial is that both clinician and client agree to test a treatment and then the client is randomized to receive either the active treatment or the placebo. Following a period of time on one treatment, the client is then given the other treatment. This pair of treatments is then repeated several times where the order of the treatments is randomized. For trials of drug treatment, both the patient and the clinician are blind to which treatment is being given. The important clinical outcomes are monitored, usually by some form of patient diary until the prearranged end of the trial has been reached or the clinician and patient are convinced that the active treatment is effective, harmful, or has no effect. Interpretation of the outcome of the trial is usually by straightforward visual inspection of the diary or graphs plotted from it. An alternative approach is to use some simple statistical tests, usually a paired t-test. Guyatt et al[1] have described their experience of providing an N of 1 service to a university hospital where they found that 84% of completed trials provided a clear answer to a clinical question. The main reason for not completing an N of 1 trial, which occurred in 18% of trials that started, was patient or clinician noncompliance. Mental health problems that they were involved in included anxiety and psychosis.

Guidelines for completing an N of 1 trial (adapted from Guyatt et al.[2] with permission from Canadian Medical Association)
Is an N of 1 trial indicated?

Treatment factors
Is the effectiveness of the treatment really in doubt? Here we need to be sure that large randomized controlled trials of the treatment have not been done by searching the literature. If large trials have been done we need to assess their relevance to the patient. Other treatment factors which would indicate an N of 1 trial is needed would be disagreement between the clinician and patient about the merits of a particular treatment and disagreement or uncertainty about the cause of symptoms which may be attributed to a therapy.

Will the treatment, if effective, be long term? N of 1 trials are useful for chronic conditions where treatment is likely to be for long periods. Where the condition is short-lived, it is unlikely that the effort of doing an N of 1 trial is justified.

Is the patient willing to collaborate and is the trial ethical? N of 1 trials are a collaborative process between client and clinician. The patient needs to understand the process and be willing to take part. There are also ethical and legal issues here. N of 1 trials sit between the worlds of clinical and research work where they employ a research technique in a clinical setting. One way of thinking about N of 1 trials is that they are like a special diagnostic procedure that requires written informed consent. However, it would be wise to check with local ethical bodies to discover their interpretation of this. A further issue is that of patients who are under a mental health act. Here, there should be other safeguards and, while such clients should have the right to be offered N of 1 trials, local mechanisms need to be put in place to ensure that any such trials are done in an ethical way.

Is an N of 1 trial feasible?

Does the treatment have a reasonably rapid onset? Treatments which produce noticeable effects only after several months are unlikely to lend themselves to N of 1 trials. This is because of the time taken to complete any trial of treatment. In mental health, trials of different mood stabilizers for bipolar disorder would probably come under this heading.

Does the treatment stop acting soon after it is withdrawn? The most straightforward treatments to test are those which stop working when they are withdrawn. This is because they have a short washout period, which makes the trial feasible to complete in a reasonable time.

Does the treatment lead to a permanent change in the disorder? Treatments which produce permanent change in the underlying disorder are unlikely to be suitable for an N of 1 trial. Here, the removal of the treatment is unlikely to lead to an immediate return to pretherapy levels of symptoms. This is a problem for several psychotherapies and physical therapies. However, some variations on the N of 1 trial describe having prolonged baseline periods between treatments so that treatment effects decrease before the introduction of the next therapy.

Can clinically important outcomes be measured? Symptoms may be measured by their severity, for example the amount of pain or degree of depression, or by their frequency, for example the number of panic attacks or binge-eating episodes per week. Alternatively, outcomes may be measured for example, by their effect on functioning, days worked, or tasks completed. Usually outcomes are recorded by the client in some form of diary, which may be daily or weekly. Similarly, side effects of treatment may also be recorded.

How long should the trial run for? This can be decided in advance, especially if there is going to be some statistical testing of the results. Alternatively, if there is a marked difference in response between the two periods, the clinician and patient may want to stop the trial after just one pair of treatments. If the difference is not marked, then it is recommended that at least two pairs of treatments are completed before the trial ends.

Is the trial feasible in my practice?

Is there a pharmacist or researcher who can help us? For drug trials, collaboration with a pharmacist is important. Pharmacists may be able to prepare the placebo, do the randomization and perhaps measure compliance. For nondrug trials, collaborating with a researcher who is familiar with single-subject experimental designs can be useful.

Do we need help interpreting the data? In practice, the most feasible way of interpreting the data is by visual inspection of the outcome data. If more sophisticated analysis is required to assess the role that chance could have played in the outcome, then performing a paired t-test seems the simplest way to proceed. Some clinicians and patients may enroll statistical help at this point.

Reports of N of 1 trials in the literature for mental health problems include the treatment of depression by methylphenidate in a patient with AIDS[3] and the use of the same drug in treating attention deficit hyperactivity disorder (ADHD) in school-aged children.[4] In the latter study fifty families with children who had been diagnosed with ADHD were each entered into an N of 1 trial of three weeks where they were given a placebo for one of the weeks and two different doses of methylphenidate for the other two weeks. Outcomes were measured by parents and teachers at baseline and the end of each week. The teachers, parents, and the clinicians did not know the order of medication for each child. At the end of the three weeks about three-quarters of the children had responded to the methylphenidate, two-thirds of whom took the drug long term. Probably more important was the feedback from the families, all of whom indicated that taking part in an N of 1 trial had helped them make a decision about treatment. In the AIDS trial, an outpatient with mild depression was treated with two weeks of methylphenidate and two weeks of placebo. Neither patient nor clinicians were aware of what the patient was taking until after the trial. Outcomes were measured of mood and cognition, the mood symptoms by the Hamilton Rating Scale for Depression and a mood self-assessment scale, and cognition by digit span, trail making tests, and the symbol digit modalities test. It was concluded that for this patient methylphenidate did help with the depression but only improved some cognitive tests. In both these examples, the patients were willing to take part, the effect of the treatment was in some doubt, and it was planned to take the medication for some time if it was effective. Methylphenidate is a medication which acts quickly but doesn't appear to alter the underlying condition in depression or ADHD. The outcomes were important and easily measured by the patients and their families in both trials.

Decision analysis

Decision analysis, originally developed in the business world[5] is an explicit, quantitative approach to examining difficult decisions where there is uncertainty about the outcome. This may well be the case where there is little evidence available on which to base a decision. It may also help identify gaps in the research literature; produce protocols for patient management which clinicians may use in audit and teaching; involve the patient in management; enable the clinician to ask hypothetical questions; and provide an alternative way of evaluating new treatments and investigations by incorporating widely dispersed research findings. There have been few published examples of its use in mental health.[6–10]

The technique involves several discrete steps:[11] defining the problem, structuring the problem by drawing a decision tree, estimating the probabilities and values of various outcomes, and then analysing the tree. We have chosen an example involving the decision to offer prophylactic mood stabilizing treatment postpartum to a 28-year-old woman with a history of bipolar disorder (with thanks to Dr. Susan Jackson for this example). The patient had a history of two manic episodes in her early 20s followed by two depressive episodes. She described the manic episodes as a 'terrifying experience'. This was her first pregnancy and when we first broached the idea that she may be at risk of relapse following the birth of her baby she was shocked, initially not believing that she could relapse. She rang around her social network, including friends with medical knowledge, and felt very anxious around making the decision. Her response when she returned to us was that she found it very difficult to weigh up the variables in the choice she had to make and asked us to summarize the information for her. We decided to apply decision analysis to this problem to see if it could be useful.

Step one: defining the problem

First we had to break the problem into its separate parts. We had to identify what choices had to be made, for example which treatments she could be offered, and what possible outcomes may realistically arise. For the patient, she had to weigh up the possible benefits of taking a mood stabilizer to prevent a relapse against the advantages and disadvantages of breastfeeding or not breastfeeding while taking the mood stabilizer. The choices were, firstly, prophylaxis versus no prophylaxis postpartum and, secondly, breastfeeding versus no breastfeeding. The types of prophylactic treatment open to us were lithium, sodium valproate, and carbamazepine. We chose to focus on sodium valproate as the data suggest that this is the safest of the three to use in breastfeeding. The three outcomes we were mainly interested in were recurrence of the mood disorder; adverse effects for the infant from the mood stabilizer in breast milk; and whether the child was breastfed or not.

Step two: structuring the problem

Our next task was to structure and display the components of the problem in a logical way that displays where choices must be made and where chance events occur. Such a structure is a decision tree (Fig. 11.1). In itself, this process can be helpful by making clinicians and patients pay attention to all the different outcomes – especially when it comes to the order in which they perform tests or treatment. By convention where there is a choice of action (a 'decision node') a square is used and where the outcome is decided by chance (a 'chance node') a circle is

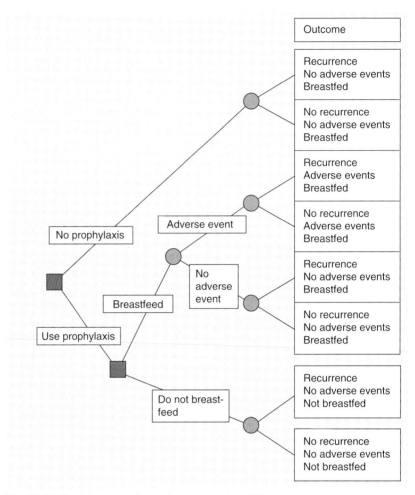

Fig. 11.1 Decision tree for using a mood stabilizer postpartum.

drawn. In this case, the decision nodes represent a choice between using a mood stabilizer versus not using a mood stabilizer and, secondly, whether to breastfeed or not. The circles represent the points where the patient may suffer a recurrence of her mood disorder and where the infant may suffer adverse effects from the drug in her breast milk.

Step three: estimating the uncertainties and the value of the different outcomes

For each chance node we needed to assess the probabilities of the different outcomes. We can do this by reference to the literature or by using best guesses. This can often be a useful exercise to highlight why different clinicians and patients make different decisions with the same information. One person's unlikely may be another person's common. For the outcomes, we need to assign each a relative value; this is often referred to as its 'utility'.

To estimate the uncertainties in this decision, we need to know, firstly, what are the chances of someone with a history of bipolar disorder relapsing postpartum with and without a mood stabilizer and, secondly, what is the probability of an infant suffering an adverse event if sodium valproate is present in the mother's breast milk. We searched the literature and in the time available the most relevant paper we could find was by Cohen et al.[12] that looked at the risk of relapse in women with a history of bipolar disorder treated with lithium and carbamazepine during the first 48 hours postpartum. One of 14 women (7%; 95% confidence interval 0% to 33%) treated prophylactically relapsed in the three months postpartum compared to 8 out of 13 (61%; 95% confidence interval 36% to 85%) who were not treated. (Of the five women in the second group who did not relapse, two went on to receive prophylaxis in the first three weeks postpartum.) Unfortunately, this paper did not include sodium valproate as a mood stabilizer, but a quick look at the literature on mood stabilizers reassured us that in terms of efficacy the three main mood stabilizers seem to be equivalent. (One of the advantages of decision analysis is that we can check how important this assumption is in making the decision about treatment.) Secondly, we searched the literature to find out the risk to the infant of exposure to sodium valproate in the breast milk. In Medline, we could not find anything which referred to newborn babies, but we did find a study which followed up 110 children with a mean age of 4 who were taking sodium valproate. This showed that 8% of children over the two years of follow-up had to discontinue treatment due to side effects, usually nausea and vomiting. There were no serious side effects in this group, but also no discussion of the potential long-term effects of treatment in infants who are less able to metabolize the drug.

Step four: generating the utilities/ranking the outcomes

The next part of a formal decision analysis is to find out what value to place on the different outcomes. By this stage in the analysis, you and the patient may have already clarified things enough to make a decision. However, where there is still uncertainty or dispute, especially between different members of the same team, this step can be helpful. The different outcomes are given a ranking between 0 and 1, with 1 being the best outcome and 0 the worst with the other outcomes lying in between. In this scenario, the best outcome is for there to be no recurrence, no adverse events in the baby, and for the baby to be breastfed – this is given a value of 1. The worst outcome is that the patient has a relapse of her illness, and the baby suffers an adverse event from the drug while being breastfed – this is given a value of 0. For the intermediate outcomes, probably the best way to assign a value to them is to use a 'basic reference gamble'. Here, the patient (or whoever is assigning a value to the different outcomes) is told that they are facing two doors, A and B. Behind door A they will definitely get one of the intermediate outcomes, in this case a relapse of their illness but no adverse effects in the baby who is breastfed. If they choose door B they have a 50% chance of the best outcome and a 50% chance of the worst outcome. They are then told they have to choose one of the two doors (Fig. 11.2).

The probabilities of the chances of getting the two extremes are then changed and the patient is again asked to choose between the two

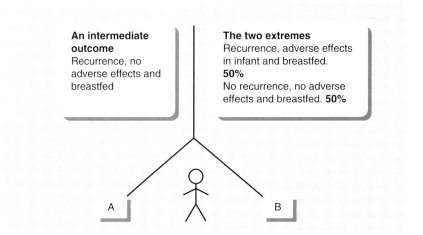

Fig. 11.2 The basic reference gamble.

doors. This is repeated until the patient can no longer make a choice – this is the 'point of indifference'. At this point the probability of the best outcome behind door B is the utility of the intermediate outcome behind door A. When we did this gamble with the patient, she gave the following utilities to these outcomes:

- No recurrence, adverse effects in infant, breastfed = 0.35
- Recurrence, no adverse effects in infant, breastfed = 0.30
- No recurrence, no adverse effects in infant, not breastfed = 0.9
- Recurrence, no adverse effects in infant, not breastfed = 0.1

We also went through this process with the key worker and found that she placed a much higher value on nonrecurrence of the mood disorder and less emphasis on the value of breastfeeding the baby.

Step five: analysing the decision tree

The utility values and the probabilities are now added to the decision tree (Fig. 11.3), and the utilities for each chance node calculated. The utility of each final outcome is multiplied by the probability which immediately precedes it, and at each chance node these new utilities are added together. If a chance node branches into one or more other chance nodes, the utility at the next chance node on the right is used in the sum. This process is called folding back the decision tree. For a decision node, the best choice is that with the highest utility at its first chance node.

For the patient, the best choice here would be to use prophylactic medication and not breastfeed the baby (this is the chance node with the largest outcome utility of 0.951). However, one of the advantages of decision analysis is that the assumptions behind decisions can be manipulated to see how much difference they make to the final choice. Using the 95% confidence limits from the studies quoted above, we could alter the probability of relapse on and off medication to see if this

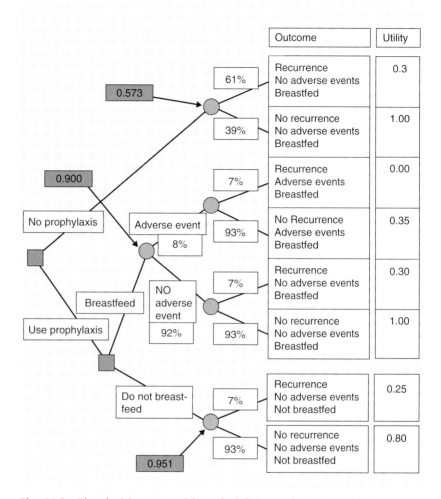

Outcome	Utility
Recurrence No adverse events Breastfed	0.3
No recurrence No adverse events Breastfed	1.00
Recurrence Adverse events Breastfed	0.00
No Recurrence Adverse events Breastfed	0.35
Recurrence No adverse events Breastfed	0.30
No recurrence No adverse events Breastfed	1.00
Recurrence No adverse events Not breastfed	0.25
No recurrence No adverse events Not breastfed	0.80

Fig. 11.3 The decision tree with probabilities and utilities added.

changes the decision. We can also see from this that even though we have assumed a relatively high incidence of adverse effects in the infant if exposed to sodium valproate, changing this to lower values is not going to make much difference to the outcome. What the patient decided to do in the end was to take the minimum effective dose of sodium valproate from day 1 postpartum and to breastfeed the baby, which would have baseline bloods, regular monitoring, and be under pediatric care. We also emphasized other methods to reduce stress and maintain sleep. Although this was not the best outcome (0.900 versus 0.951) the patient chose it for two reasons. Firstly, when we altered the probabilities of relapse on prophylaxis to the extremes of the confidence intervals, that is the chance of relapse on medication increased from 7% to 33%, then this in fact did become the best option. Secondly, she felt a lot more informed and comfortable with this decision having been through the decision analysis process. Other advantages of this process were that it encouraged a review of the literature; highlighted where data is lacking and suggested where future data could be collected; highlighted the different values held between the patient and the key worker; and was easy to modify and adapt once the structure was in place.

Criticisms of decision analysis

Traditional clinic decision making, using clinical 'rules' and intuition, can be criticized because of its often unrecognized implicit assumptions.[13] Decision analysis, however, is often criticized because of its explicit assumptions.[14] The criticisms follow the basic stages of decision analysis.

Defining and structuring the problem

A common critique of decision analysis is that problems are defined too narrowly and do not replicate clinical practice – there are not enough choices and not all the possible outcomes are considered.[15] While this may be true of some analyses, it is not insurmountable. Indeed, defining the problem and deciding upon the important outcomes, and where the clinician has to make choices can be sufficient in itself to solve it.

Assigning probabilities

The probabilities drawn from the published literature or from clinicians 'best guesses' may be inappropriate or nonexistent. However, intuitive decision making faces the same problem when the database is inadequate. Clinicians may find it difficult to quantify their estimates of probability – one doctor's 'very likely' may be 90%, another doctor's 75%. An advantage of decision analysis is that sensitivity analysis allows change of these estimates to judge how important individual differences are. Also, clinicians' personal probability estimates may explain why they make different decisions in similar circumstances.[16]

Assessing relative values or utilities

There are three main difficulties with this.[17] The first is the process of quantifying imprecise outcomes, – for example the value of being pain free. Converting these into numbers may be difficult, but no more so than when rating scales convert emotions such as depression into numbers using standardized rating scales.

Second is that most outcomes have multiple attributes. An outcome such as 'recurrence but no side effects' is made up of many different factors including the severity of any symptoms, the time off work, economic cost, the stigma of psychiatric contact, and effects on family functioning. Ransohoff & Feinstein[17] argue that all these different outcomes should be given separate utility values, which are then expressed on a single scale. The objection to this view is that people can assign relative values to outcomes without doing the same for their individual parts. For example, most people would be able to decide on the relative merits of travelling by train or car without also having to list the relative merits of the economic and environmental costs, convenience, and comfort. Decision analysis may be criticized for making this process explicit, but any other model of decision making – including 'normal clinical practice' – also has to find a way of ranking different outcomes.

The third objection to assigning utilities to outcomes is who should do it – the patient, doctor, or society? Each of these decision makers could place different values on the same outcome. Rather than being a drawback, this is an advantage of decision analysis. It helps to highlight ethical dilemmas where the needs of the individual have to be balanced against the needs of society and the duties of professionals.

There are other difficulties in obtaining utilities. The way in which doctors frame questions affects the response of the patient.[18] The effect depends on whether the patient views a particular outcome as a loss or a gain, for example whether the question is about survival or mortality. In addition, utility values may not be consistent over time or changing circumstances. How people's utility values change when they are ill is not known. However, an advantage of decision analysis is that sensitivity analysis may answer such 'what if' questions.

Analysing the decision tree

A problem here is how to interpret differences between the final expected utilities. Should clinicians give the same weight to the difference between 0.1 and 0.2 as they do to 0.5 and 0.6? Brett[19] has pointed out the ethical dilemmas of decision analyses designed for groups of patients that produce small differences in the final utilities. Such analyses, by seeking the greatest good for the population, may 'sacrifice' individuals who were destined to do well without treatment.

A final criticism of decision analysis is that it is not clinically useful. Sackett[20] quotes a figure of 1:80 routine admissions where he used decision analysis. Plante et al.[21] performed between 14 and 40 consultations a year over seven years, three-quarters of which were formal decision analyses by a clinical decision consultation service. They do not present any data on the impact the service had on patient care, an area for future research.

In psychiatry, many situations are unique to one patient, so any analysis may be difficult to 'export' to other patients. Hamm et al.[22] suggest other problems. Structuring the decision tree is difficult when patients may not always make rational choices and where the doctors' actions may be constrained by the law. The probabilities that apply in unique situations may be difficult to measure, especially when the decision maker affects the actions of the patient. In these circumstances, the probabilities of events are not independent of the choices made by the clinician.

There are situations where these objections do not apply and decision analysis may prove useful, for example in a conflict over management in a multidisciplinary team. Worrall[23] describes his use of a decision tree in resolving conflicts between doctors over the use of electroconvulsive therapy as well as in teaching, and Bonner[10] has used it to describe the nursing decision-making process regarding putting a patient under the mental health act in a community setting. However, a major difficulty with decision analysis is that it is time consuming for busy clinicians.

For these reasons, we believe that it will be most useful when developing pathways for common difficult situations where utilities may be 'plugged into' decision trees which have previously been developed.

Some of these trees may be published and the following critical appraisal rules adapted from Sackett[24] may help in their assessment.

Critical appraisal of studies on decision analysis

Are the results of a decision analysis valid or true?

1. Was the decision tree clinically sensible; that is, were all the important outcomes and treatments included?
2. Were the range of probabilities of the outcomes valid and credible?
3. Was the derivation of the utilities clearly described in a way which you could use in your situation?
4. Was their a sensitivity analysis (that is, were the probabilities) altered to reflect the effect of extremes on decision making?

Are the results of the decision analysis important?

1. Was there a clear outcome so that one choice of action led to a significantly higher utility?
2. Was this choice of action consistent across a range of different credible probabilities and utilities?

Are the results of the decision analysis relevant?

1. Do the probabilities apply to our patient?
2. Can our patient, family, or health professional state their utilities in a useable form?

What this chapter does is to provide you with some alternatives to relying on clinical 'instinct' when faced with problems for which there is little evidence for their solution.

References

1. Guyatt GH, Keller JL, Jaeschke R, et al. The N-of-1 randomized controlled trial: Clinical usefulness. Our three-year experience. Annals Int Med 1990; 112:293–299.
2. Guyatt GH, Sackett DL, Adachi JD, et al. A clinician's guide for conducting randomized trials in individual patients. Can Med Ass J 1988; 139:497–503.
3. White JC, Chistensen JF, Singer CM. Methylphenidate as a treatment for depression in acquired immunodeficiency syndrome: an N-of-1 trial. J Clin Psychiatry 1992; 53(5):153–156.
4. Kent MA, Camfield CS, Camfield PR. Double-blind methylphenidate trials: practical, useful, and highly endorsed by families. Arch Ped Adol Med 1999; 153(12):1292–1296.
5. Moore PG, Thomas H. The Anatomy of Decisions. London: Penguin; 1988.
6. Hatcher S. Decision analysis in psychiatry. Br J Psych 1995; 166:184–190.
7. Schulberg H, Block M, Coulehan J. Treating depression in primary care practice. An application of decision analysis. Gen Hosp Psych 1989; 11:208–215.
8. Koenig H, Ford S, Blazer D. Should physicians screen for depression in elderly medical inpatients? Results of a decision analysis. Int J Psych Med 1993; 23:239.
9. Dantchev N. Decision trees in psychiatric therapy: review. Encephale 1996; 22:205–214.
10. Bonner G. Decision making for health care professionals: use of decision trees within the community mental health setting. J Advanced Nurs 2001; 35(3):349–356.
11. Weinstein M, Fineberg HV. Clinical Decision Analysis. Philadelphia: WB Saunders; 1980.
12. Choen LS, Sichel DA, Robertson LM, Heckscher E, Rosenbaum JF. Postpartum prophylaxis for women with bipolar disorder. Am J Psych 1995; 152(11):1641–1645.

13. Tversky A, Kahneman D. Judgement under uncertainty: heuristics and biases. Science 1974; 185:1124–1131.

14. Feinstein AR. Clinical biostatistics XXXIX. The haze of Bayes, the aerial palaces of decision analysis, and the computerised Ouija board. Clinical Pharm Ther. 1977; 21:482–496.

15. Dolan JG. Can decision analysis adequately represent clinical problems? J Clin Epid 1990; 43:277–284.

16. Schwartz WB. Decision analysis. A look at the chief complaints. New Eng J Med 1979; 300:556–559.

17. Ransohoff DF, Feinstein AR. Is decision analysis useful in clinical medicine? Yale J Biol Med 1976; 49:165–168.

18. McNeil BJ, Pauker SG, Sox HC, et al. On the elicitation of preferences for alternative therapies. New Eng J Med 1982; 306:1259–1262.

19. Brett AS. Hidden ethical issues in decision analysis. New Eng J Med 1981; 305:1150–1152.

20. Sackett DL, Haynes RB, Guyatt GH et al. Clinical Epidemiology: a Basic Science for Clinical Medicine. 2nd edn. Boston: Little, Brown and Co; 1991.

21. Plante DA, Kassirer JP, Zarin DA, et al. Clinical decision consultation service. Am J Med 1986; 80:1169–1176.

22. Hamm RM, Clark JA, Bursztajn H. Psychiatrists' thorny judgements. Describing and improving decision making processes. Med Decision Making 1984; 4:425–447.

23. Worrall EP. Consent to treatment and clinical decision analysis. A solution to medical uncertainty and public doubt. Psychiatric Bulletin 1989; 13:79–81.

24. Sackett DL, Straus SE, Scott Richardson W, et al. Evidence-Based Medicine. How to Practise and Teach EBM. 2nd edn. Edinburgh: Churchill Livingstone; 2000.

12

Putting it all together – practicing evidence-based mental health care

The original emphasis of evidence-based health care was on critical appraisal and solving clinical problems. However, few clinicians have the skills and more importantly the time needed to do this routinely. There are also practical problems to accessing information in a timely manner. The change in focus is that now clinicians are more frequently being presented with critically appraised evidence so that the main task involves questions relating to importance and relevance. It is also clear that the knowledge, skills, and attitudes inherent in the practice of evidence-based health care are useful in several areas of a clinician's professional practice. We have listed some uses of evidence-based health care below (Box 12.1) and will describe them in more detail in this chapter.

Managing yourself

EBM as an ethical issue

We have found that the most important step in using the ideas from evidence-based health care in self management is convincing yourself and others that it is an important clinical skill. A key aspect here is the difference between practice and learning. Often these are differentiated so that learning, of which evidence-based practice is a part, is seen as a luxury to be indulged in when there is time. However, our view is that evidence-based health care incorporates both practice and learning and that it is probably unethical not to do it. It fits in with a model of lifelong learning and the principles of transparent maintenance of professional standards in health care. This is reflected in the demands for all health professionals to have in place a system of credentialing. Relevant here is that learning is not a rational process but affected by unconscious strong feelings. Adults learn less well than children, especially more senior clinicians (who are supposed to be fully grown up), who may be particularly anxious about not knowing or not being an expert. Exposure of need, the sense of not knowing, and loss of cherished ideas

> **Box 12.1**   Uses of evidence-based mental health care
>
> - As a tool for managing yourself – developing a reading habit and for maintenance of professional standards (MOPS)/continuing professional development (CPD).
> - As a way of managing the culture of multidisciplinary teams.
> - For solving clinical problems.
> - For teaching, including journal clubs.
> - For deciding how to allocate resources.
> - For 'evidence-based' consultations with patients.

about competence can precipitate infantile feelings of paranoia and hostility often seen in clinicians and masked as rationalization – not enough time, support, or skills – which can be significant barriers to successful learning.[1]

How to build evidence-based practice into continuing professional development – what works and what does not work

What does not work is clear. Traditional continuing medical education (CME) for doctors does not work as an educational tool, although it may be very important for maintaining networks and morale. A systematic review of continuing education practices found that interactive continuing medical education with the opportunity to practice skills could change professional practice and occasionally health care outcomes. Didactic lecture sessions do not appear to be effective in changing behaviour.[2] Other approaches with some evidence of success are audit and feedback,[3] which appear to have small to moderate effects, and academic detailing or educational outreach programs.[4] For both of these interventions, the evidence is strongest on their effects on prescribing, probably because this is relatively easy to measure. Their effects on other health care behaviors have not been thoroughly tested. Interestingly, the effective approaches are rooted in the individual clinician's personal experience so are directly relevant to practice. Here, the skills and knowledge of evidence-based health care are important in answering questions around the importance and validity of what is learned.

Developing a reading habit

Practitioners in training and those in established posts have different needs for reading. Trainees have to keep exams in mind and also read background information on the disorders they treat (for example, fundamentals of psychopharmacology or the basics of behavioral therapy). For this reason we think that developing an effective reading habit is harder for trainees than for established professionals who (hopefully) will have done the background reading and be in a post where the types of problems they see are reasonably predictable.

Developing a reading habit involves two steps – first, deciding what to read and, second, how to manage the habit. Deciding what to read is relatively straightforward. Given that there is so much information available on mental health care, we need to develop some rules around what we read and probably more importantly what we do not read. Clinicians need to decide first what journals they will regularly scan for potentially useful articles and then, within those journals, what articles to read. Deciding what journals to read depends partly on feasibility – what is available and affordable. Within what is feasible, clinicians can choose journals which are specific for their interests as well as journals which deal with wider health care issues, such as the *BMJ*, *JAMA* or the *Lancet*, all of which often contain important information on mental health care. Trainees, will have to read more widely than colleagues who have completed training and will need to select from journals with a wider scope, such as the *British Journal of Psychiatry* or the *American Journal of Psychiatry*. Deciding what articles to read in each journal usually involves the application of the critical appraisal questions for each particular paper. As the critical appraisal guides are hierarchical it is usually feasible to decide whether to read an article or not by applying the first guide for each type of paper. For example, for articles about the effectiveness of therapy, if the subjects were not randomized to a treatment and comparison group, then it is probably not worth investing your precious time in reading the paper. (This does not mean the study is worthless, just that if you have only a limited amount of time to read to keep up with the literature you have to invest your time in reading articles whose conclusions may have some validity – 'power reading' in other words.) Fortunately, there are now at least two publications which do the screening and critical appraisal of articles for clinicians. These are *Evidence-Based Mental Health* and *Evidence-Based Nursing*. Both journals screen over 100 relevant journals for high-quality articles which, when they are identified, are critically appraised with a commentary. *Evidence-Based Mental Health* is published quarterly by the BMJ Publishing Group Ltd, The Royal College of Psychiatrists, and the British Psychological Society (*http://ebmh.bmjjournals.com/*). It is multidisciplinary with a target readership of psychiatrists, psychologists, nurses, social workers, occupational therapists, pharmacists, and other health professionals involved in mental health care. *Evidence-Based Nursing* is published by the BMJ Publishing Group and the Royal College of Nursing Publishing Company and is also published quarterly: (*http://ebn.bmjjournals.com/*). While it is not specifically directed towards mental health, it often contains relevant articles. You can arrange with both of these journals for them to automatically send their most recent contents page to your e-mail.

Keeping up to date electronically is possible in two main ways (*http://www.sacme.org/Research/keepinguptodate.htm* The Society for Academic Continuing Medical Education website). Firstly, an increasing number of journals will, like the evidence-based journals, send you their table of contents (TOC) regularly by e-mail. Secondly, there are alerting services for either Medline or the Internet. The alerting services automatically send you updates of new literature or relevant articles from the web. You sign up with a provider (often this is free), indicate what you are interested in, and then the alerting service regularly scans Medline or the Internet for relevant information, which it then automatically informs you of. The difficulty with most of these is that the information is rarely critically appraised before you get it, and there is also the problem of being overwhelmed with updates that you never get round to reading. One alerting service we particularly like is PubCrawler ('It goes to the library. You go to the pub'. *http://www.pubcrawler.ie/*) This is a free alert service for PubMed and GenBank, created by the Department of Genetics, Trinity College, Dublin. It scans the daily updates from these databases and lists new entries that match users' research interests. We used PubCrawler for writing this book. One of us put 'evidence-based medicine' in as a search term and every week PubCrawler sends us the citations to the most recent entries in Medline that have been indexed under this medical subject heading. (Note: it does not send the whole article, just the reference.)

Having decided what to read, the hard part is managing yourself to actually do it. This involves deciding when to read, where to read, how to keep a record of what you have read and designing a storage and retrieval system that works for you. Doing this successfully involves applying the principles of behavioral therapy to ourselves. In particular, we should set SMART goals, that is goals that are specific, measurable, achievable, realistic, and timely. Firstly, where to read. Most clinicians we know take home articles to read and use time at weekends and in the evenings to catch up on their subject. We think that this is the wrong approach, for several reasons. Firstly, it is not looking after ourselves or modelling what we should be telling our clients about boundaries between work and nonwork activities. Secondly, if we accept that reading to stay current is a core clinical skill and is important for our patients, then it should be given an equal status to other activities and done in work time. Hiding away core activities like this in nonwork time ensures that they are not resourced or supported adequately. Lastly, and probably most importantly, is allocating time to reading. Most clinicians overestimate how much time they read about their subject each week. Generally, the more senior the clinician the less time they have each week to read. There is no substitute for writing time for reading in a diary, in other words booking time with yourself for continuing professional education. Writing things down is important and makes it much more likely that things will happen. After all, this is how most outpatient clinics (and behavioral therapies) work. It is also important that other people in your team know that this is time for keeping up to date. Keeping a record of what you have read is relatively straightforward and can be done in a separate continuing professional education diary, a hand-held computer, or a notebook. The important thing again is that progress and what you have done is written down. Having a system of storage and retrieval is harder. Probably the most useful for you and your patients is to enter appraised data and references into a hand-held computer that you use at work. This way you can build up a library of valid, important, and relevant articles specifically for yourself that is accessible and feasible to use. Having a paper filing system is probably best used for important background information and key papers used in teaching. It seems to us too great an effort to try to produce a separate system parallel to the local library. Headings in a paper filing system could be MeSH headings to make it consistent with Medline (although in our experience this can lead to rapidly multiplying subheadings with only a few papers under each heading) or, as one of us does, using the chapter headings from a standard textbook for file headings.

As a way of managing the culture of multidisciplinary teams

Introducing an evidence-based culture into organizations is more than teaching individuals critical appraisal skills. It involves paying attention to strong feelings of resistance to any change as well as providing leadership and technical support. The technical solutions of organizations introducing 'knowledge systems' and developing information systems are straightforward.[5] In practice, as with all change in complex organizations, what is equally if not more important are issues of leadership and strong feelings that resist change. These feelings can be even stronger around issues to do with learning, as we have described above. Newman et al.[6] describe the introduction of evidence-based nursing practice into an NHS ward. They encountered a variety of responses including non-participation by members of staff who worked part-time, nights, or had worked on the ward for many years; enthusiastic uptake by nurses as part of an academic project; and the ward manager acting as a negative role model who was supportive of the project but failed to fulfil her commitments to it. There was also, as is usual in health care, continuing change in other areas including changes in the nursing assessment process of patients, changes in the ward environment, and so on. Despite all this, the documentation of patient care improved and the number of sick days per month amongst nurses reduced by 10 days from the same period in the previous year. Participants in the project reported that their confidence had increased. This reflects our own experience in that having an evidence-based culture gives clinicians alternative tools to wrestle with the clinical problems they encounter. This gives us a language for addressing problems that we would not otherwise have and with this common language (which transcends professional backgrounds) we can promote team discussion and cohesiveness. The teaching of students, of whatever clinical discipline, using the language of evidence-based mental health care, also promotes this.

As well as the teaching of evidence-based skills to practitioners, there is the challenge of implementing evidence-based practice in routine clinical settings. How to do this well is still not clear and is the main issue in producing clinical guidelines – it is not what is in them but how they are disseminated and implemented that is the key issue. One group which is evaluating this process is the US National Evidence-Based Practices Project which aims to implement effective mental health practice in different settings in the US.[7] The researchers in this project describe several key issues in implementation: first, that education alone is ineffective; second, that change occurs over time; third, that stakeholder involvement is important; and lastly, programs are likely to work if they match the values, needs, and concerns of practitioners.

Teaching and journal clubs

As we alluded to in the previous section, teaching at the clinical coal face is an important stimulus for introducing evidence-based ideas and promoting an evidence-based culture. Teaching may take the form of educational prescriptions[8] or may be encouraged in other ways. At the University of Auckland, medical students in their clinical years have to do Critically Appraised Teaching Topics (CATTs) as part of their assessments during their clinical years. These are presented to the teams they are allocated to and help to encourage an evidence-based culture.

For more senior clinicians there is the traditional journal club, sometimes melded together with a case conference. The first journal club was described by Sir William Osler at McGill University in 1875 and was for the purchase and distribution of periodicals he could not afford to subscribe to alone. The goals of journal clubs since then have changed so that they are now important for teaching critical appraisal skills and for encouraging attendees to develop a reading habit. They are also important social occasions where senior clinicians, trainees, and other professionals can meet regularly. Organizational factors which seem to be effective in running a journal club are primarily having a designated leader who 'owns' the management of the journal club, plus participation by senior clinicians and clear educational goals.[9] Specific teaching of critical appraisal skills can incorporate the presentation of a clinical scenario, formulation of a question important to the patient, and then critical appraisal of an article as it relates to the client.

For deciding how to allocate resources

How to allocate health care resources will always be a contentious and difficult area. Like clinical decision making, it involves evidence but also values and other resources. While some see evidence-based care as 'scientific rationing', it seems to us to provide a useful, shared language to have sensible conversations with funders about setting priorities. One area where this has been done with some controversy and varying degrees of effectiveness has been the American Psychological Association's Division 12 (Clinical Psychology) Task Force on the Promotion and Dissemination of Psychological Procedures.[10] This task force produces a short list of treatments which meet the criteria for 'well established' and 'probably efficacious', which clearly has implications for funding. The work was extended in 1999 in Hawaii to childhood and adolescent mental health conditions. The controversy centered around the presence of behavioral and cognitive therapies in the list, to the exclusion of other psychological therapies. This was partly due to the fact that these therapies are the most amenable to randomized controlled trials and that the people entering such therapies are often easier to categorize that clients receiving other therapies such as psychodynamic treatment. This has exacerbated the tensions between cognitive behavioral practitioners and the 'humanistic practitioners'.[11] The fear is that these lists could be used by funders in the US to restrict payment to treatments which only appear on the list. So far, the evidence that this is happening is minimal. It has also led to a healthy debate about what sort of evidence could demonstrate the effects of humanistic therapies and what information do policy makers need to make decisions about funding. The English and Welsh NHS seems to have gone down this route with a model of evidence-based psychotherapy practice that includes efficacy and effectiveness evidence, acknowledges what psychotherapies have in common and focuses on the quality of service delivery.[12]

For solving clinical problems and 'evidence-based' consultations with patients

Evidence-based health care has been 'sold' to clinicians as a way of solving clinical problems. It is certainly a useful tool in this regard. Solving clinical problems can also be built into a reading habit and teaching. It does not necessarily provide an answer to all clinical problems but it does describe part of a process for arriving at a decision. Difficult clinical decisions have clinical, ethical, and legal dimensions, and the techniques of evidence-based health care inform the clinical dimension. Like most difficult decisions, there usually is not a 'right' answer, but there is a correct process for arriving at a decision.

An interesting question to ask is 'how does an evidence-based mental health consultation differ from a nonevidence-based consultation?' One answer is that research evidence is explicitly incorporated into the conversation. This would involve referring to research when making decisions about treatments as well as answering questions about etiology, prognosis and related questions. However, as we have pointed out previously, the integration of evidence-based care into patient consultations is one of the areas which has been least researched. A type of consultation where the ideas of evidence-based practice could clearly be used is in making decisions about treatment where risks and benefits have to be explained and understood. While the epidemiological emphasis has been on the type of numbers to include in the conversation (NNTs for example), there is also considerable evidence from the psychological literature that clients' decisions can be influenced by how questions are framed. Framing risks positively (for example, chances of survival) is more effective than negative framing (for example, chances of death) in getting people to make risky choices. Giving patients more information of any sort, however framed, makes them more wary about accepting any tests or treatment. To counter this, it is better to express risks in both negative and positive frames; to avoid the use of relative risk; to make comparisons with everyday risks; and use graphical representations of risk.[13] We have previously described in the chapters on treatment and decision analysis various ways in which clinicians can elicit patients' and other key individuals' values when it comes to making treatment choices. We suspect that this area of evidence-based health care will be a growth area of research over the next few years. It is right and proper to end on this note, as we have tried to emphasize that evidence-based health care, like this book, begins and ends with patients.

References

1. Taylor D. Emotional factors and continuing professional development. Advances in Psychiatric Treatment 2001 (7) 9–15.
2. Davis D, Thomson O'Brien MA, Freemantle N, et al. Impact of formal continuing medical education: do conferences, workshops, rounds and other traditional continuing education activities change physician behaviour or health care outcomes? JAMA 1999; 282 (9):867–874.
3. Thomson O'Brien MA, Oxman AD, Davis DA, et al. Audit and feedback: effects on professional practice and health care outcomes (Cochrane Review) In: The Cochrane Library, Update Software. Issue 1, 2003.
4. Thomson O'Brien MA, Oxman AD, Davis DA, et al. Educational outreach visits: effects on professional practice and health care outcomes (Cochrane Review) In: The Cochrane Library, Oxford: Update Software, Issue 1, 2003.
5. Tomlin A, Dearness KL, Badenoch DS. Enabling evidence-based change in health care. Evidence Based Mental Health 2002; 5:68–71.
6. Newman M, Papadopoulos I, Melifonwu R. Developing organisational systems and culture to support evidence-based practice: the experience of the Evidence-Based Ward Project. Evidenced-Based Nursing 2000; 3:103–105.
7. Torrey WC, Drake RE, Dixon L, et al. Implementing evidence-based practices for persons with severe mental illnesses. Psychiatric Services 2001; 52:45–50.
8. Sackett DL, Strauss SE, Richardson WS, et al. Evidence-Based Medicine. How to Practise and Teach EBM. 2nd edn. Edinburgh: Churchill Livingstone; 2000.
9. Dirschl DR, Tornetta P, Bhandari M. Designing, conducting and evaluating journal clubs in orthopaedic surgery. Clin Ortho and Rel Res 2003; 413:146–157.
10. American Psychological Association. Task Force Reports on Empirically Supported Treatment, Division 12 Central Office, PO Box 1082, Niwot, CO 80544, USA.
11. Elliott R. A guide to the empirically supported treatments controversy. Psychotherapy Research 1998; 8:115–125.
12. NHS Executive. NHS psychotherapy services in England: review of strategic policy. London: Department of Health; 1996.
13. Edwards A, Elwyn G, Mulley A. Explaining risks: turning numerical data into meaningful pictures BMJ 2002; 324:827–830.

Appendix A

Antidepressants for depression in medical illness (Cochrane Review)

Gill D, Hatcher S

ABSTRACT

A substantive amendment to this systematic review was last made on 22 August 2000. Cochrane reviews are regularly checked and updated if necessary.

Background: Depression in the physically unwell is common and an important cause of morbidity. There are problems with diagnosing depression in the physically ill which may lead to under-recognition and under-treatment. In clinical practice antidepressants are available and a feasible option for treating depressive disorders. Therefore we thought it would be a reasonable first step in addressing this problem to describe the literature of randomised controlled trials in this area.

Objectives: To determine whether antidepressants are clinically effective and acceptable for the treatment of depression in people who also have a physical illness.

Search strategy: MEDLINE, Cochrane Library Trials Register and Cochrane Depression and Neurosis Group Trials Register were all systematically searched, supplemented by hand searches of two journals and reference searching.

Selection criteria: All relevant randomised trials comparing any antidepressant drug (as defined in the British National Formulary) with placebo or no treatment, in patients of either sex over 16, who have been diagnosed as depressed by any criterion, and have a specified physical disorder (for example cancer, myocardial infarction). 'Functional' disorders where there is no generally agreed physical pathology (e.g. irritable bowel syndrome) were excluded. The main outcome measures are numbers of individuals who recover/improve at the end of the trial and, as a proxy for treatment acceptability, numbers who complete treatment.

Data collection and analysis: Data was extracted independently by the reviewers onto data collection forms and differences settled by discussion.

Main results: 18 studies were included, covering 838 patients with a range of physical diseases (cancer 2, diabetes 1, head injury 1, heart 1, HIV 5, lung 1, multiple sclerosis 1, renal 1, stroke 3, mixed 2). Depression was diagnosed clinically in 3 studies, otherwise by structured interview or checklist.

Only 5 studies described how they performed randomisation. 1 study compared drug with no treatment, and the rest with placebo: all of the latter said they were double blind.

6 studies used SSRIs, 3 atypical antidepressants, and the remainder tricyclics.

Patients treated with antidepressants were significantly more likely to improve than those given placebo (13 studies, OR 0.37, 95% CI 0.27-0.51) or no treatment (1 study, OR 3.45, 95% CI 11.1-1.10). About 4 patients would need to be treated with antidepressants to produce one recovery from depression which would not have occurred had they been given placebo (NNT 4.2, 95% CI 3.2-6.4).

Most antidepressants (tricyclics and SSRIs together, 15 trials) produced a small but significant increase in dropout (OR 1.66, 95% CI 1.14-2.40. NNH 9.8, 95% CI 5.4-42.9). The 'atypical' antidepressant mianserin produced significantly less dropout than placebo.

Only 2 studies used numerical scales designed to measure effects on function and quality of life; in HIV (Karnofsky scale), drug was better than no treatment; in lung disease (Sickness Impact Profile), drug was not significantly different from placebo.

Only 7 studies reported looking for changes in the physical disease. Antidepressants produced no change in immune function in HIV relative to placebo (2 studies) or no treatment (1 study). Relative to placebo, antidepressants produced no change in cardiovascular function in heart disease, in respiratory function in lung disease, or in vital signs or laboratory tests in cancer (1 study each). Nortriptyline produced worse control in diabetes.

Trends towards tricyclics being more effective than SSRIs, but also more likely to produce dropout were noted, but these are based on non-randomised comparisons between trials.

Reviewers' conclusions: The review provides evidence that antidepressants, significantly more frequently than either placebo or no treatment, cause improvement in depression in patients with a wide range of physical diseases.

About 4 patients would need to be treated with antidepressants to produce one recovery from depression which would not have occurred had they been given placebo (NNT 4.2, 95% CI 3.2-6.4).

Antidepressants seem reasonably acceptable to patients, in that about 10 patients would need to be treated with antidepressants to produce one dropout from treatment which would not have occurred had they been given placebo (NNH 9.8, 95% CI 5.4-42.9).

The evidence is consistent across the trials, apart from 2 trials in cancer, where the "atypical" antidepressant mianserin produced significantly less dropout than placebo.

Trends towards tricyclics being more effective than SSRIs, but also more likely to produce dropout were noted, but these are based on non-randomised comparisons between trials.

Problems with the evidence include most of the trials' use of observers, rather than patients, to decide on improvement, and concentration mainly on symptoms rather than function and quality of life. There is also a possibility of undetected negative trials.

Nevertheless, the review provides evidence that use of antidepressants should at least be considered in those with both physical illness and depression. Regarding diagnosis, the existence of a cheap and readily available treatment for depression should encourage detailed assessment of persistent low mood in the physically ill.

Citation: Gill D, Hatcher S. Antidepressants for depression in medical illness (Cochrane Review). In: *The Cochrane Library*, Issue 4 2002.

Appendix B

Example of a Medline record

UI - 22106160
PMID-12112158
DA - 20020711
DCOM-20020821
IS - 0885-6230
VI - 17
IP - 7
DP - 2002 Jul
TI - Prophylactic therapy with lithium in elderly patients with unipolar major depression.
PG - 619-22

AB - OBJECTIVES: To compare the relapse rate of elderly depressed patients taking low dose lithium as an additional therapy with antidepressant medication to those receiving antidepressant medication alone. METHODS: Fifty elderly subjects recovering from a major depressive illness taking continuation antidepressants were randomised, in a double blind study, to receive additional lithium carbonate or placebo and followed up over a two year period for evidence of relapse. RESULTS: Relapse rate was significantly greater in those subjects taking antidepressant medication alone compared to subjects taking additional lithium therapy. After six months four (17%) subjects taking antidepressant medication alone had relapsed, whereas none of the subjects taking additional lithium had relapsed. After two years eight (33%) subjects taking antidepressant medication alone had relapsed, whereas only one (4%) of the subjects taking additional lithium had relapsed. CONCLUSION: This preliminary study suggests that long-term low dose lithium therapy is well tolerated and protects elderly patients from a relapse of depressive illness.
CI - Copyright 2002 John Wiley & Sons, Ltd.

AD - MARC, Elderly Mental Health Directorate, Moorgreen Hospital, Southampton. Dwilk2000@aol.com
FAU - Wilkinson, David
AU - Wilkinson D
FAU - Holmes, Clive
AU - Holmes C
FAU - Woolford, Janet
AU - Woolford J
FAU - Stammers, Susan
AU - Stammers S
FAU - North, Janine

AU - North J
LA - eng
PT - Clinical Trial
PT - Journal Article
PT - Randomized Controlled Trial
CY - England
TA - Int J Geriatr Psychiatry
JID - 8710629
RN - 0 (Antidepressive Agents)
RN - 554-13-2 (Lithium Carbonate)
SB - IM
MH - Aged
MH - Antidepressive Agents/adverse effects/*therapeutic use
MH - Depressive Disorder/*prevention & control
MH - Double-Blind Method
MH - Drug Therapy, Combination
MH - Female
MH - Human
MH - Lithium Carbonate/adverse effects/*therapeutic use
MH - Male
MH - Recurrence/prevention & control
MH - Statistics, Nonparametric
MH - Support, Non-U.S. Gov't
EDAT-2002/07/12 10:00
MHDA-2002/08/22 10:01
AID - 10.1002/gps.671 [doi]
PST - ppublish
SO - Int J Geriatr Psychiatry 2002 Jul;17(7):619-22.

Appendix C

Steps in conducting a systematic review

Procedure	Elements
Formulate the review question	A well-constructed question should include four elements: • The target population • The intervention(s) • The comparison(s) • The outcome(s) of interest
Define inclusion and exclusion criteria	These should be defined *a priori* and include criteria for: • The participants in the studies • The intervention(s) • The comparison(s) • The outcome(s) of interest • The types of study design to be included and other methodological quality features to be considered
Identify studies	Define a search strategy with the aim of identifying all relevant studies (both published and unpublished). The search strategy should include: • Searches of major electronic databases using predefined search algorithims • Handsearching of key journals • Checking of the bibliographies and reference lists of identified relevant studies • Checking of conference proceedings of relevant conferences • Direct contact with researchers who are active in the field • Search of thesis and dissertation databases
Select study	Relevant studies will be selected or excluded on the basis of the predefined criteria. To ensure this process minimizes bias: • Eligibility should be checked independently by two assessors • There should be a predefined procedure for resolving disagreements about eligibility • A log of the excluded study and reasons for exclusion should be maintained
Assess study quality	The methodological quality of each study should be assessed on the basis of predefined criteria. To ensure this process minimizes bias: • The quality of each study should be rated by more than one assessor • The assessors should be blind to authors, institutions, and journals of the studies

(Continued)

Appendix C   Steps in conducting a systematic review – Cont'd

Procedure	Elements
	For systematic reviews of controlled trials there should always be assessment of: • Concealment of treatment allocation • Blinding • Handling of patient drop-out
Extract data	The extraction of data and forms for entry of the extracted data should be planned and piloted before commencing the actual data extraction. It is preferable that: • Data extraction is undertaken by more than one assessor • The assessors should be kept blind to authors, institutions, and journals
Analyse and present results	• The results from individual studies should be tabulated • A graphical representation (such as a forest plot) of the results should be undertaken • A statistical test for heterogeneity should be undertaken and, if present, the studies should be carefully examined for the possible sources of heterogeneity • Meta-analysis of all the studies or subgroups of studies might be undertaken • Sensitivity analyses might be undertaken to determine if the findings are robust and not unduly sensitive to certain assumptions or decisions made by the researchers • A list of excluded studies should be made available to the readers
Interpret results	The researcher(s) should: • Consider and discuss the limitations of the review • Consider the strength of the evidence • Consider applicability and generalizability • If possible, provide a numeric interpretation of the results, which is understandable to the readers • If possible, consider economic implications • Consider implications for future research

(Adapted from Egger M, Davey Smith G, Altman DG. Systematic Reviews in Health Care. Meta-analysis in context. London: Blackwell Publishing; 2001, with permission.)

Index

Chaos in dynamical systems